The
Food Allergy
Book

*The foods that cause you pain
and discomfort and how to
take them out of your diet*

The Food Allergy Book

*The foods that cause you pain
and discomfort and how to
take them out of your diet*

William E. Walsh, M.D., F.A.C.A.

with contributions by
Felicia Busch, M.P.H., R.D.

ACA Publications, Inc.
St. Paul, Minnesota

International Standard Book Number 0-9631544-7-8
Library of Contress Catalog Card Number 94-96717

Designed and Composed by Barbara Field

ACA Publications, Inc.
1690 University Avenue West, Suite 450
St. Paul, Minnesota 55104
Tel: 612/649-3523   Fax: 612/649-3509
Toll free: 1-800-649-3523

Printed in the United States of America

Contents

Preface

When we go on a journey, we expect to complete it safely and at our destination. Unfortunately, that doesn't always happen. Think of the poor passengers on the Titanic who paid their money to enjoy the maiden voyage of this luxurious ocean liner, content in the knowledge that the ship was virtually unsinkable. Unfortunately, this bold claim made no impression on the iceberg that brought their voyage to disaster.

Fortunately, most of the time our journeys end safely and we reach our destination, usually with the help of a few key people. For instance, if you were going to Germany you might first visit a travel agent, an expert in trip planning. To get to the airport you call a cab; the driver is an expert in city transportation. You board a plane whose pilot is an expert in flying. You stay in a hotel staffed by experts in lodging. Your trip goes smoothly because competent experts handle each step.

A book is like a journey for your mind. You read it because you have a destination or goal you want to reach; when you finish, you hope to have reached this goal. If the book is a detective story or science fiction novel, you want excitement and entertainment; from a biography or wildlife novel, you desire knowledge and adventure. From a medical book, you hope to gain the most precious knowledge of all, a way to improve your health.

That is the purpose of this book. I hope that when you complete your journey through its pages, you gain a little knowledge to ease the problems life makes you face. And just as you have every right to question the qualifications of the people who help you on your make-believe trip to Germany, you have every right to question my qualifications, since I am your travel guide, cabby, and pilot on this trip. Let me give them to you.

I am a medical doctor with the same M.D. degree as a pediatrician, family doctor, or internist. After completing medical school, I served two years in the U.S. Air Force, where I had the opportunity to care for an allergy clinic. The field of allergy fascinated me, and I realized I would be happy spending my life treating people with allergy problems; I also realized that the field is so complicated I needed further training. As I think back to those days, I know I was right in both cases. I am happy treating people with allergy and I'm glad I sought further training to put me on firmer ground in this demanding field.

This training was obtained at the Mayo Clinic, where I spent four hard-working but enjoyable years. The clinic, through its expert teaching staff and diverse patient load, offers the allergist-in-training magnificent opportunities to study the many areas he or she is responsible for when treating people, areas such as allergic dermatology, allergic chest disease, allergic gastrointestinal disease, and many others, as well as how pollen, dust, and mold affect patients with allergy.

After completing my training at the Mayo Clinic, I moved to St. Paul, Minnesota, in 1970, where I started my current allergy practice. Shortly afterward, I took and passed an examination certifying me as a specialist in allergy. The certificate is from the American Board of Allergy and Immunology and is recognized by the American Board of Pediatrics and the American Board of Internal Medicine.

The American Board of Allergy and Immunology sponsors active programs to keep allergists up to date, including providing the opportunity to retake the test at specified intervals, a process called voluntary recertification. To ensure that my knowledge remained current, I took the recertification exam in 1980 and again in 1990, on each occasion earning my recertification diploma.

I have described my credentials to assure you that the book you are reading was written by a qualified medical doctor who tries to stay current with modern scientific knowledge of allergic illness. Although the training and diplomas are essential to making a medical book credible, they are only part of the reason this book exists. Equally important are several other factors.

One factor is perhaps most significant because it makes me uniquely qualified to write this book. I share with many people a great susceptibility to the harm caused by foods. Perhaps that's understandable; who wouldn't be fascinated by a medical illness if they were its victim? I know my medical problems steered me toward my specialty in the first place, and I remember how it happened.

I was walking to work on a lovely fall day in 1965, looking quite nice in my spiffy Air Force captain's uniform. But my mind wasn't on enjoying the warm, green Nebraska scenery; instead my thoughts twisted and turned as I considered the many specialized fields of medicine my M.D. degree unlocked. Which one for me? Should it be Family Medicine, which brings with it the satisfaction of caring for all the illnesses of my patients, of being the first doctor they call when they are ill? Or maybe Obstetrics, for the joy of delivering healthy babies? Or perhaps Plastic Surgery, for the pride of restoring a ravished face? Or Psychiatry, with its awesome potential for working with the human mind and emotions?

Then the obvious struck me, and I stopped and laughed. There I was, standing in a green and weedy field at the height of the fall ragweed pollen season, my eyes running like a crying baby's and my nose dripping like old plumbing with a leak, wheezing like a couch potato running a marathon. To add to my miseries, my armpits were itching from contact dermatitis caused by sensitivity to a deodorant. I said to myself, "Bill, whatever could you be other then an allergist?"

I have never regretted that decision, and as I pick up new allergies, they serve to reinforce and renew my interest in, and fascination for, the field of allergy. When foods began to trouble me, my attention to food allergy increased enormously, especially when articles in the allergy literature started questioning whether allergists paid enough attention to patient's complaints about food. I discovered I paid little attention, and I resolved to change.

Eating when hungry, drinking when thirsty, and making resolutions are equally easy; growing food in a drought, finding water in a desert, and keeping resolutions are equally hard. However, because of my own food reactions, keeping my resolve to study food allergy was easy. Unfortunately I found treating food allergy uncommonly difficult. Why? Because my patients told me about food reactions that the allergy literature said weren't supposed to happen, reactions to foods the literature said didn't cause symptoms. In fact, because my patients' stories of their food allergies contradicted the allergy literature, I was becoming more and more confused and frustrated.

That I needed to learn about food allergy was obvious; what was not obvious was where this knowledge existed. I was forced to choose between accepting the allergy literature's view of food allergy or believing my patients when they told me their weird-sounding stories of food reactions. I chose to believe my patients.

I'm glad I did. Over a period of years, their strange tales started to make sense, a pattern of reactions emerged, a dietary approach was born. I wish I could say the diet sprang from my brilliant deductions, but that's not true. My patients taught me the diet a little at a time as they related their discoveries about the foods that aggravated their headaches, hives, and diarrhea. Each discovery lessened the confusion surrounding food allergy; each discovery added another important element to the diet.

Which brings me to why I wrote this book. I wrote *Treating Food Allergy, My Way* for several reasons, but the first and most important reason is my patients. I wrote it for them. I am so very proud of them.

The poker game of life dealt them a miserable hand, full of headaches, stuffy noses, wheezing, skin itchiness and rashes, abdominal discomfort, achiness, tiredness, and other illnesses. Many people with similar tribulations gave up and stopped trying to find a way to conquer these illnesses. They accepted their pain and misfortune, using the comforting blanket of self-pity to soothe their distress. Not my patients. They did not give up.

Although knowledgeable people—including some doctors—tried to discourage them from finding the reasons for their distress, they never stopped looking. The search brought them to my office and ultimately to the dietary changes that form such a large part of their treatment.

By their perseverance, they amply demonstrate their determination. They are not quitters. I think they are heroic. In the first edition of the book, I did not adequately express this thought. With this revision, I hope to correct my oversight.

I wrote this book to better explain the foundation of our diet and to help guide my patients through the many dietary choices they must make each day. Many have told me it does that. However, I keep hoping that I can explain these choices better. If so, my patients will have more useful knowledge about which choices are most appropriate. To help them gain this knowledge, I rewrote sections of the book, striving to more clearly guide my patients as they eat at home and in restaurants.

Although this book was written to guide those we treat, others who are not our patients have read it and found it helpful in controlling their burdensome illnesses. This is good.

As my sympathy extends to the patients who have sought our help, it also extends to those who will never come to our office for treatment. How many people in various walks of life are suffering because they are unaware that allergy induces their pain and discomfort? I hope this book helps them. If it does—if people I will never meet gain relief from their food-caused illness—I will be pleased. Their health is a reward that gives me great delight.

Acknowledgments

This book and the diet it describes would not exist without the help of many contributors. I am honored to acknowledge this help and to thank those whose generous assistance was so essential.

Much of the dietary advice contained in this book is new and surprising and was originally discovered, not by me, but by patients observant enough to recognize the foods and beverages responsible for their illnesses. These novel aspects of the diet became permanent additions when other patients found they were important in controlling their symptoms.

To those patients whose insights shaped the diet and to those patients who followed the diet and confirmed its value, I extend a heartfelt thank you. It would never have been developed without your counsel and guidance.

Just as the help of my patients was essential in developing this diet, so was the assistance of the nurses who work with me. Each is a registered nurse who has specialized for many years in the care of the allergic patient. My nurses and I approach the treatment our allergic patients as a team, from their initial evaluation and diagnosis through their followup care. I want to express my gratitude to each member of that team: Shirley Hess, Arleene Nietz, Corinne Peterson, Jan Ryan, and Caryl Steenberg.

To my patients' pediatricians, family physicians, and internists, my heartfelt thanks. These dedicated men and women comfort my patients when the are sad, care for them when they are ill, and bring the benefits of modern medicine to their bedsides. Without them, my practice would not be possible.

I am also grateful for the fine work and cooperation of Felicia Busch. Her expertise in the food sciences considerably enhances the value of this book for the food-sensitive person, and this expertise is readily apparent on examination of her practical advice on following the diet.

Many others have contributed to the diet and the book, including Barbara Field, whose skills with writing helped make sense of many murky passages. To all of you, my deepest thanks.

WILLIAM E. WALSH

The case histories described in this book are representative of many conversations with patients who have similar illnesses and food allergies. They are included to help the reader understand food allergy and its treatment. Although the essence of each case history is preserved, the names, occupations, and certain facts have been changed to prevent recognition of the patients and protect their privacy.

The Key

Were you ever out walking alone, late at night, the wind blowing icy needles of rain against your face, the darkness closing in around you? Chilled and uncomfortable, your imagination populates the night with vague and sinister demons. An uneasiness lurks at the edges of your consciousness, a wariness that raises the hair at the back of your neck, a sensation that you're being watched. At last you see the familiar sight of home, a safe haven with its bright lights and warm, dry rooms smiling a welcome that says, "Come in and I will give you comfort and protect you from the dark night." With a great feeling of relief you reach into your pocket and find—no key! You are left out in the cold, damp night.

Such is the importance of a key in our lives; it allows us to enter locked places that assure us warmth and protection. A key is equally important in our thinking. A branch of knowledge may be as elementary as the techniques used in digging a hole or as esoteric as the formulas used in flying to the moon. But whether simple or complicated, the process of thinking depends on certain key facts so important that if they were missing, the branch of knowledge would be reduced to confusion and uncertainty.

And so it is with medicine. Over the centuries many areas of medicical knowledge advanced dramatically when certain key facts became known. Just think of the wonderful heart, lung, and kidney transplants performed today—procedures previous generations of doctors couldn't even imagine—or the fantastic antibiotics that routinely kill germs that used to send us to the grave. Truly remarkable advances due to the discovery of a few key facts.

Unfortunately, not all areas of medicine have experienced such dramatic advances. One area of medical knowledge that has made little gain is the science of food allergy. Food allergy remains mired in confusion and uncertainty because the scientists who study it and the doctors who treat it are missing a crucial piece of information—information so vital that without it, treatment usually ends in failure. In this book we will examine that key piece of information, how a remarkably common group of foods and beverages can cause so many illnesses in so many people.

How To Use This Book

Don't Try To Make This Book Your Doctor

The purpose of this book is to tell you about the way I treat food allergy. I hope to alert you to some of the foods and beverages that cause my patients' symptoms—they may also hurt you. If so, and if you avoid them, I hope you will stop hurting. I did not write this book to tell you how to diagnose these illnesses. This diagnosis must be done by your primary doctor, who may be a family doctor, pediatrician, or internist. That is their specialty.

In my allergy practice, I try to make sure each of my patients has a primary doctor who has already diagnosed allergy and excluded—as far as possible—nonallergic illness as the cause of my patients' symptoms. If you were my patient and we questioned the cause of your illness, I would send you to your primary doctor for diagnosis. Go to him or her now if there is any question about your diagnosis. Don't try to guess your diagnosis by reading this book.

If your doctor wants help in diagnosis, he or she may suggest you see a neurologist, dermatologist, or other specialist; if so, for heaven's sake, take this advice. Don't try to make this book your diagnostic specialist.

Maintain a Healthy Diet While You Follow My Dietary Advice

Some of the foods and beverages I ask you to avoid add no value to a healthy diet. Other foods and beverages are championed by dietary experts who teach us they are a necessary part of a healthy diet (a number of dieticians are scandalized that we ask our patients to exclude them). Excluding these foods and beverages is not fatal to a healthy diet. There are plenty of healthy foods you can eat while you follow my diet.

In certain circumstances, there is a danger you will slip into a nutritionally inadequate and therefore unhealthy diet. For instance, if you already follow a medically pre-scribed diet that excludes healthy foods, and you also try to exclude the foods and beverages that trouble my patients, your diet may be inadequate and your health threatened. The same threat could surface with a diet not prescribed by a doctor. *If there is any chance your diet will become inadequate and unhealthy, do not follow my diet until you consult your doctor or a dietician.*

Why

As humans, we become uneasy and irritated when forced to follow instructions and we don't understand why. Who can blame us for this desire for knowledge, this demand to have *why* explained to us. Perhaps it is this curiosity about reasons, which prompts our irritation when we are ignorant, that distinguishes humans from animals. (In distinguishing humans from animals, it sometimes helps to have clues.)

I know I share this desire to know why. When I began to realize the complexity of food allergy, it became apparent that my patients would be forced to avoid a surprising number of foods and beverages, and I didn't have any idea why this was so; what made these seemingly different foods and beverages cause the same misery? The foods and beverages are different—orange juice differs from diet pop and cheese is not the same as soy sauce—but they are also similar in their effects. Orange juice, diet pop, cheese, and soy sauce all cause the same headaches or hives or diarrhea. I was learning how to treat my food-sensitive patients, but I was not learning why my treatment worked. I was irritated and frustrated.

The Usual Explanation of Food Allergy

There is an explanation of food allergy that is widely accepted by allergists. All animal- and vegetable-derived foods are made up of proteins, fats, and carbohydrates. Many of the food proteins are identical to our own body's protein, and the allergic person absorbs and digests them with no difficulty. But some proteins are different. They are only found in such foods as shrimp or nuts or cows' milk. The body does not recognize them, and in the allergic person these strange proteins lead to trouble.

When even a tiny amount of the strange shrimp, nut, or milk protein gains entrance into the allergic person's bloodstream, it is grabbed by an antibody called IgE. This antibody alerts the body to the presence of the strange protein, and the body reacts alarmingly. It releases chemicals that welt the skin in hives, clamp down on the small air passages in the lungs, causing wheezing, and the large air passages, causing choking, and dilate the blood vessels, dropping the blood pressure and threatening shock and unconsciousness.

This is an irrational overreaction to a harmless protein, like shooting a mosquito off your leg with a shotgun. Unfortunately, the allergic person is stuck with it.

My patients were not describing this sort of food allergy. Their symptoms weren't quick, striking, and dramatic; they were chronic and persistent. Also, tiny amounts didn't set off symptoms, only excess amounts—overloads. And proteins weren't involved. Our concepts of food allergy did not fit. I was confused.

A New Type of Food Allergy

Then I recalled some principles of biochemistry I learned in medical school and an explanation became apparent. I don't know if the explanation is correct, but I think it is; I know it helped me understand why my patients need to avoid certain foods and beverages.

To understand the explanation, it helps to compare your body's cells to miniature cities. They are special cities, not at all like our present-day metropolises that use coal, oil, and natural gas for power. Instead, the cell cities in our bodies use a miracle fuel as powerful as nuclear fuel but without many of the dangers associated with nuclear power plants. (That's obvious! Have you ever heard of a cell with lead or cement shielding?)

This marvelous fuel has to be handled carefully. Instead of being shoveled or pumped into a furnace to be consumed by fire all at once, it goes through a series of furnaces, each furnace releasing energy to the cell by burning only part of the fuel. When the last furnace is done, the remaining fuel is renewed by adding special chemicals, and the whole cycle of energy production starts again. A complicated process to produce power, but tremendously efficient.

Because this energy-producing process is complicated, it needs to be controlled. In our make-believe world of the cell city, this control is achieved using methods like those of our real cities; a bureaucracy rules. Let's look at this bureaucracy.

The bureaucrats are surprisingly alike. As children they were pudgy; their classmates called them Fats or Wart or Bumble; they were the type of student who told the teacher, "The homework assignments are due today," and they never got dirty. They were perfect children, although a tad slow in their thinking, a mite short on creativity, and a bit lacking in flexibility. Anything out of the ordinary flustered them and led to confused inactivity.

As adults, the bureaucrats still are surprisingly alike. Their fellow rulers call them Robert, Alexander, and William (their exaggerated sense of importance allows no nicknames). They are pudgy, pompous, and persnickety, and good administrators as long as everything is going well; but any disruption causes disaster. You see, they are still a tad slow in their thinking, a mite short on creativity, and a bit lacking in flexibility. The bureaucracy of the cell city is unlike that of our modern society, where flexibility, creativity, and clear thought are so necessary and practical.

An old expression tells us that into every life a little rain must fall. Unfortunately for our bureaucrats, rain can turn to a flood. The problem arises from another group that populates our little cell city—an antibureaucratic group. A group of rebels.

Markedly different from the bureaucrats, this second group went by the nicknames of Sly, Speed, and Flash as youngsters; their names fit their mischief. They never finished their homework on time, so when the little bureaucrats reminded the teacher the assignments were due, they seethed with anger.

Sly, Speed, and Flash and their friends thought fast, found creativity a snap, and were utterly flexible. Unfortunately, they were also little devils. If there was trouble brewing, they were first in line. If teacher sat on a pin, their pleas of innocence rang through the room. If someone tripped a little bureaucrat, they were guilty. Engaging little chaps, but in their bodies not one grain of responsibility.

As adults, they are just as fast-thinking, creative, and flexible, and just as lacking in responsibility. Their delight and pleasure in life is to torment the bureaucrats, and they know a perfect way to achieve this fiendish goal. You see, this fantastic energy production can only work if the fuel, which is hot and corrosive, is slowly and precisely transported to the furnaces (one of the few virtues of the bureaucrats is their precision—and they are slow). Our rebels delight in sending extra trainloads of fuel to the furnaces, where they dump it all over the floor.

You can imagine what happens next. Our poor bureaucrats, faced with this mess, call out the National Guard and enlist workers from factories and offices to shovel up the corrosive goo. This makes everybody unhappy. The

National Guard is grumpy because the gooey fuel eats through their shiny boots. The office and factory workers hate the backbreaking work and their union strikes in protest, closing the assembly lines, supermarkets, and sales organizations of the little cell city. The city grinds to a halt, the voters complain, the mayor screams, the bureaucrats are reduced to quivering ineptness. It's a real mess.

Pity the poor bureaucrats. Slow-thinking, lacking creativity and flexibility, they are unprepared for this major disaster. After undergoing psychiatric treatment for acute anxiety, induced by the disruption in their precious orderliness and the upheaval in the city they rule, they slowly and ploddingly restore the energy-producing system to normal and restart the offices and factories. And calm the mayor and soothe the voters. And wait for the next onslaught of excess fuel for the furnaces.

The Moral of the Story

Perhaps you think the story of the little cell city is preposterous? Are you saying to yourself, "No way is that story a model of the cell"? If these are your thoughts, you are wrong.

What We Know

The marvelous material that stores the energy of the atom without the dangers of its radioactivity is sugar. The analogy of the furnaces is a good one; sugar slowly releases its fantastic energy, a bit at a time, as if it were traveling from furnace to furnace. In biochemistry books, this process is called the Krebs cycle or the tricarboxylic acid cycle.

The counterparts of the bureaucrats in the body are the enzymes that precisely regulate sugar's energy release. Made of proteins, the prime function of these tricky molecules in energy production is to regulate and assist in the splitting of the sugar molecule that releases energy. Without them, sugar would need furnace heat to split, making life impossible unless we were built like your home furnace. (Imagine dating someone who looks like your furnace!)

So the furnace-like production of energy actually takes place in the body; because it is regulated by enzymes, there is no need for furnace heat. Enzymes do fantastic work, but don't be fooled. They are not creative or flexible or quick thinking; they ploddingly and persistently perform the limited tasks to which they are assigned.

What I Believe To Be True

To continue the explanation, you must accept the rest of the story as I see it and believe it to be true.

It is tempting to look at our modern world, to see computers, bullet trains, and swept-wing fighter planes, and to conclude that not only has the world changed, we've changed. In some ways, perhaps we have. But not our bodies nor our cells.

The last thousand years have brought profound changes in our lifestyle. However, a thousand years is a tiny moment in the evolution of our bodies, of our cells. They are the same cells our ancestors possessed in the ancient past, in a cave, crowded close to a fire. In fact, they are not much changed from that monkey-like creature whose descendants walked upright and learned to talk. We share the same nutrition needs, digestion limits, and energy production method.

What has changed is our diet, specifically our use of refined foods. Prior to modern agriculture, foods were made of unrefined protein, starch, and fat. We all know the ponderous impact of refined fats on our bathroom scales.

Starches are made of sugar molecules, tightly bound together like links on a chain. In digestion, the individual sugars are snapped off the chain slowly and ploddingly, allowing lots of time to process each sugar and insert it into the energy production system. No hurry, everything orderly. The bureaucratic control of energy is content.

Proteins are like starches, chains of amino acids that are broken off the chain slowly, ploddingly, and contentedly.

Refining starches and proteins produces regrettable consequences. Refining breaks the bonds between sugar molecules so the sugar you eat and drink enters the stomach no longer in chains. The molecules are like the links of a busted chain; they are free. The body gobbles up this unchained sugar like a hungry shark in a goldfish aquarium. Unfortunately, although our digestive system can regulate its intake of sugar from starch, it has inadequate ability to regulate its intake of refined sugar. Conditioned by millions of years of evolution to handle a diet of starches, its enzymes do not have the flexibility and creativity to adapt to a diet high in refined sugar.

The refined sugar floods the body, causing the various systems that process sugar to overload. What happens then is unclear, although I like my fanciful explanation of the little cell city and the havoc that overload causes. I believe it has illness-causing effects, and I hope to further explain this belief in other sections of this book.

Before ending this chapter, a word about proteins. The story is much the same as with sugar. Refining breaks apart the linked amino acids that make protein. The free amino acids gush into the body, overwhelming the amino acid handling systems. The body suffers harm.

What Is Allergy?
What Is an Allergist?

Most of us became familiar with the word *allergy* as young children, either because we ourselves had an allergic reaction such as hives or eczema, or one of our siblings or friends had allergies. In other words, our understanding of allergy is based on what it *does* to people rather than what it *is*. However, before we can understand what an allergist is, we will need a more precise definition of allergy.

What Is Allergy?

Allergic illness arises from the body's sensitivity to the pollen, dust, mold, food, and certain other substances we are exposed to in the environment. Why does the body react? Because it mistakes things free of harm for things full of danger.

For instance, a harmless bit of ragweed pollen meanders by, minding its own business, not a nasty thought in its tiny mind. For some odd reason, the nose reacts fearfully to contact with this innocent pollen, rushing into frenzied activity—sneezing, dripping, itching, and stuffing up—as if the pollen were intent on starting a horrible infection. It's not—the nose is mistaken. Unfortunately, the miserable person attached to the nose suffers.

It is the same with food allergy. The wretched person affected by this process eats a little shrimp and disaster strikes. His eyes water, his body swells, he chokes as his air passages close, and his skin grows a crop of red splotches as if a heavenly painter has spattered him with barn paint. Again, a mistake in identification. The body thought the shrimp was an attacking enemy. Most uncomfortable and definitely dangerous. (It's beyond me why the body defends itself by almost killing itself!)

Pollen, dust, mold, and food do not directly cause any allergic symptoms. They are triggering mechanisms, just like the trigger on a gun. The bullets they release are numerous natural body chemicals, some with familiar names such as histamine, others with improbable names like the slow-reacting substance of anaphylaxis. These chemicals flood the body, dilating blood vessels, leaking fluid, itching nerve fibers, and, in general, making a horrible mess. They stuff the nose and hive the skin when we allergic people encounter ragweed, shrimp, and the numerous other things that cause allergies.

The Scope of Allergy

That a patient is suffering from an allergic illness is sometimes quite obvious. It may strike dramatically and quickly—the sneezing and swollen eyes after contact with ragweed and cat dander are obvious, as are the acute hives and choking after eating shrimp. The diagnosis is often confirmed by blood tests that measure an antibody, called IgE, which attaches to the ragweed, cat dander, or shrimp. Usually the skin tests are positive, again confirming the diagnosis. These reactions are within the scope of allergy.

But the allergic basis of some illnesses is not obvious. These illnesses don't strike suddenly; they develop slowly. No IgE antibody against the cause floats in the bloodstream; a skin test answer doesn't magically appear in thirty minutes. However, they also fit within the scope of allergy—they are caused by the same environmental exposures and foods that bring on the more easily recognized sudden symptoms.

Patients often fail to realize that their discomfort and pain are caused or influenced by allergy if the symptoms develop slowly, symptoms such as headache and asthma and eczema, plus many others. In fact, they frequently tell me, "I would have come to see you long ago if I had known my headaches (or chronic diarrhea or chronic hives, etc.) were due to allergy."

Two Types of Food Allergy

Food allergy frequently appears in a quickly developing form where the cause is usually obvious (i.e., a shrimp reaction). It can also appear as a slow-developing illness that is hard to diagnose.

With the sudden onset type of food allergy, people are reacting to something in the diet. Usually it is a protein, one so different from a person's own body proteins that the body becomes alarmed. For instance, there are proteins in nuts, cows' milk, and shrimp that are different from the protein making up the body's muscles and internal organs. When the body recognizes this strange protein, it triggers the allergic illness—hives, asthma, hay fever, etc. Often tiny amounts of these proteins lead to dangerous and sometimes life-threatening reactions.

But foreign protein is not the only cause of food allergy. Some food chemicals that are not protein and not foreign to the body are also involved—chemicals that live in every cell in the body, chemicals essential for metabolism, chemicals necessary for life.

Tiny amounts of these chemicals do not cause harm. Only large amounts do, quantities so sizable the body can't handle them. The illnesses caused by this type of food allergy develop slowly and the patient has a hard time identifying the guilty foods.

To unravel the mystery surrounding the diagnosis and treatment of food allergy, the harm caused by excesses of these chemicals must be recognized. We will attempt to do this as we examine food allergy more closely.

The Role of the Allergist

"Well," you ask, "what is the role of the allergist? Certainly a gastroenterologist can uncover the foods that are causing cramps and diarrhea, a neurologist can investigate foods that are provoking headaches, a dermatologist can determine the foods that are inducing hives and eczema."

Yes, they can, and they should try to find them. However, an allergist possesses unique tools and training. For example, an allergist is trained in the application and interpretation of skin tests; in diagnosing food allergy, these tests are often essential.

In drafting their majestic plan for humanity's allergies, the architects forgot to limit food allergy to one food, but allowed a rascal assistant to guarantee that many patients' food allergies involve multiple foods. Unfortunately, this makes diagnosing reactions to these multiple foods difficult or impossible without the help of food skin tests. In many cases, a doctor trying to diagnose a complicated case of food allergy without the aid of food skin tests is like a traveler without a compass—lost in a fog of uncertainty. Food skin tests, the primary tool of the allergist, often help cut through the fog.

Two examples spring easily to mind. Jimmy, an eleven-year-old patient of mine, had a particularly baffling case of asthma—darned if I could figure it out. Food allergy didn't seem to be at fault because his asthma was so persistent. He wheezed every day and his asthma didn't vary with his diet. Out of frustration, and because I didn't know how else to find the cause, we skin tested him to foods, and a large wheat reaction surfaced. I couldn't believe it! In my experience, asthma due to wheat is rare. I was surprised when, on Jimmy's next visit, his father told me the test must have been correct because Jimmy wheezed every time he ate wheat. Avoiding wheat gratifyingly calmed his asthma.

Then there is Tammy, a clerk for a local department store, who had persistent hives due to multiple foods, including such traditional ones as lettuce, celery, and carrots. If they hadn't revealed themselves on skin tests, I don't know how I would have discovered them, and Tammy's skin would still be itchy and blotchy.

Many other illustrative cases tumble around in my memory, but I believe these two serve to make the point.

To complicate matters even further, not only do allergic patients have multiple food allergies, they also have multiple allergic illnesses. In my practice, that is not the exception, it's the rule. Again, a few examples to help you understand.

Jack is a twenty-five-year-old pipefitter who often works in dusty areas that make his constantly stuffy nose shut down completely. When he visits his girlfriend in her musty basement apartment, he wheezes and his eyes swell, perhaps due to the apartment's mold, or maybe to her cat. As a toddler, cramps and diarrhea made him scream with pain and his parents' nights seem to last centuries as they listened to his suffering. As an adult, he won't eat in a restaurant because he almost strangles if a careless food handler allows a little shrimp into his food. Even avoiding shrimp isn't enough. Once or twice a week some unknown foods or beverages give him cramps and diarrhea. He's really uncomfortable.

How can Jack find out about the cat, mold, and food allergies that plague him? It is inefficient and impractical to expect Jack to see an ophthalmologist for his eyes, an otolaryngologist for his nose, a pulmonologist for his asthma, and a gastroenterologist for his diarrhea and have each of them administer a separate set of skin tests. A far more sensible approach to diagnosing the causes of Jack's nose, eye, chest, and abdominal illnesses is to send him to a doctor acceptable to all these specialists—an allergist.

I don't mean to disparage the other specialists I mentioned. Each has a role to play in good patient care. When a patient has any illness, he or she should first see a primary doctor for diagnosis and treatment and be referred to other specialists if the primary doctor wants their help. When the primary doctor suspects allergy and wants help in diagnosing the allergic causes of a patient's illness, an allergist should be consulted.

But what about the patient who has only one allergic illness such as diarrhea? Perhaps the allergist's help is not so essential, and testing by the gastroenterologist would be sufficient. Maybe, but don't forget our impish assistant architect. I guess it wasn't in his plan for the allergic patient to have only one illness.

I am reminded of Mary, a fifteen-year-old who first came to see me ten years ago, accompanied by her mother Theresa. Poor Mary had daily cramps and weekly diarrhea, which we found was due to a number of common offenders, including tomato products, citrus fruits, and beef (surprisingly, because beef is rarely a cause of diarrhea). Three years later she returned with severe hay fever, which we found was caused by oak and ragweed pollen. Mary is now married with two lovely children, whom I met when she returned recently to tell me of her asthma, probably provoked by her basement apartment's mustiness.

The moral of Mary's story? There is no way to predict that a person will always have only one allergy. Mary would have felt ridiculous returning to a gastroenterologist to explore the cause of her hay fever or asthma. Returning to an allergist made more sense.

I told you about these patients, not to glorify the allergist, but to attempt to explain the allergist's role among the specialists your primary doctor may want you to visit. I view the allergist's primary function as that of an investigator into the causes of environmental and food reactions that can affect many areas of the body and involve any specialty from dermatology to pulmonology.

It is my hope that these examples will also help you understand this complicated field of allergy, which attempts the awesome task of studying the myriad environmental agents and foods that cause diverse illnesses. I say awesome task because the troublemaker assistant architect of allergy had no more pity on the *doctor* diagnosing allergy then he had on the miserable *sufferer*. Multiple environmental agents (dust, mold, pollen, animals), multiple foods, and multiple illnesses are often as difficult (and sometimes impossible) for the doctor to *diagnose* as they are for the patient to *tolerate*.

The complexity of allergy makes diagnosis difficult and, in my opinion, creates the need for the specialty of allergy—men and women specifically trained to recognize and test for the multiple illnesses caused by the environment, by foods, and as you will see later, by food additives.

Overview of Food Allergy

The ways in which people react to foods vary as much as the ways in which they comb their hair. They can react quickly and dramatically and recover equally rapidly—or become sick slowly and recover sluggishly. One food or many foods may bring pain and discomfort. The involved foods can be obvious and the patient sure of the cause, or the foods obscure and the person confused. For some, food allergies strike when they consume even a minuscule amount; others need to eat or drink a comparatively large quantity before experiencing pain and discomfort. On skin testing, the harmful foods may surface, or perversely hide their identity. Complicated for these poor people, isn't it?

Sudden, Dramatic Food Reactions

For many people, even tiny amounts of such foods as nuts, fish, peanuts, and shellfish can precipitate severe and life-threatening illnesses; because they are quick-striking and dramatic, a person's attention is immediately drawn to the food. There is usually no difficulty in determining the culprit. The only treatment for this type of food allergy is avoidance—don't eat the offending food.

An example of someone with this type of allergy is the person who dines at a nice restaurant, enjoying a delectable meal of shrimp. Suddenly his eyes swell and tears flow, his nasal passages become blocked, his skin erupts with angry red hives, and the swelling in his air passages begins to strangle him. The reaction is dramatic, frightening, and dangerous. No more shrimp!

Sometimes the severe reaction occurs during or after a meal at which many foods are eaten. If the multiple foods consumed make it difficult to identify the dangerous food, blood tests or careful skin tests to food will often unmask the offender.

Allergy to a Single Food

The quickness and severity of dangerous food reactions usually point directly to the involved food. Another aid to diagnosis arises when a person reacts to a single food. This is especially helpful when the ill effects appear shortly after the food is eaten. If you have diarrhea or hives every time you eat corn or carrots, you know where the problem lies.

Sometimes, a commonly consumed food such as wheat, or a beverage such as milk, is at fault. Because the food is eaten at every meal, it's hard to pinpoint (infrequently consumed foods are easier). If the patient has a hunch corn or milk provokes symptoms, he or she can avoid the suspect food or beverage for a week and then reintroduce it to the diet—repeatedly if necessary—and the waxing and waning of symptoms will usually confirm the suspicion. If there is still doubt, a skin test will often provide certainty.

Allergy to Multiple Foods

Now the diagnosis becomes more difficult. As the number of foods causing symptoms multiplies, the difficulty in finding these foods also multiplies. When a person eats or drinks a number of potentially harmful foods at each meal, it is easy to be confused. Although it is *unusual* for the patient with one food allergy to pursue allergy consultation, it is usually *necessary* for the patient with many food allergies to seek help.

Many examples come to mind, including Genny, a fifty-five-year-old mother of four and grandmother of three whose internist sent her to me after years of struggling unsuccessfully to treat her daily abdominal pains and crippling migraine headaches. Her symptoms began after her second child was born and often made the demanding role of motherhood a dreadful ordeal. In fact, pain often forced her to take to her bed, even when her children were small and needed supervision. She was miserable.

When we skin tested Genny her back flared with hives to every food tested—clearly she had multiple and serious food allergies. When I considered how to treat her, I admit I was discouraged. However, we pursued our usual approach to the patient with multiple food allergies: change the environment to reduce pollen, dust, animal, and mold exposures so she could have more "room" for food allergy; guide her in avoiding the worst foods and beverages; persuade her to rotate the rest of the foods in her diet frequently.

It worked! Genny returned to see me in three months with both abdominal pain and migraines markedly improved. No days spent in bed. My staff and I were delighted.

There are many people like Genny in our practice, each with his or her own pitiful tale. With each patient I worry whether I will be able to control these truly troublesome multiple food allergies; with almost all patients I find the tools of the allergist—combined with the patient's fine cooperation and hard work—bring about a pleasing reduction of miserable symptoms.

Slow-Developing Food Reactions

Now the diagnosis of food allergy becomes even more difficult. We no longer have the guidance of the fast-striking food reaction (i.e., eat shrimp, get sick immediately). To further confuse diagnosis, most of the patients in my practice with slow-developing food allergies are allergic to multiple foods with all the puzzlement that multiple food allergy introduces.

For instance, Linda is a forty-two-year-old printing salesperson who must often entertain her clients at restaurants. She never develops symptoms after dinner, but the next morning she wakes up feeling crummy. She feels bloated and her bathroom scale agrees; her cramps and diarrhea force her to stay home from the office or to try to go to work and have a miserable day; she is tired, irritable, and understandably depressed. (Anyone who wakes up feeling like Linda does would be depressed.)

Linda came to see me because she couldn't figure out why eating out caused such severe symptoms. She is a bright woman—any salesperson needs to be sharp to be successful—so it wasn't lack of mental ability that prevented her from recognizing the cause of her problem. The harmful foods were concealed because they were *multiple* and the reaction *slow*. It took hours for her suffering to begin.

Fortunately, we were able to single out the offending foods, and as long as Linda avoids them, she awakens refreshed in the morning.

Slow-developing food allergy presents further problems in diagnosis. It often perversely refuses to cooperate on the usual food skin tests, sometimes forcing us to abandon this highly useful tool. Other times the tests must be modified to search for delayed reactions (positive tests that take six to twenty-four hours to develop instead of the usual thirty minutes). These delayed tests can cause us to miss the diagnosis, and it is always hard to decide when to use them, or whether we need to modify the tests to accept, as positive, reactions different from the usual.

By now I think you have some understanding of the roadblocks we encounter in diagnosing the *slow-developing* and *multiple-food* allergies. You might think these are the last of the riddles we must solve as we unravel the mystery of a patient's food reactions. Unfortunately, you would be wrong; we haven't yet discussed the very important role of *accumulation* in concealing the foods that cause illness.

Accumulation

Most of us can identify with accumulation in the usual sense of the word. Remember that Thanksgiving dinner when you stuffed yourself until you felt like your stomach would burst? You just plain ate too much! You were horribly uncomfortable and berated yourself later for eating like a little piggy. You *accumulated* too much food and were unable to tolerate the sheer bulk in your tummy.

If you have food allergy, however, *accumulation* doesn't mean eating an amount of food so massive that your stomach is ready to burst. It means eating or drinking too much of the foods or beverages you *tolerate* poorly. Foods or beverages that won't hurt you in small quantities will bring pain and discomfort if you exceed that magic amount your body can handle.

With the quick-striking and dangerous food allergies, as well as with single-food allergies, and many times with multiple-food allergies, it takes only a small amount of food to bring illnesses. Patients can't tolerate any of the food. However, with accumulative food allergy, the patient *can* tolerate some of the food, but any quantity above this tolerance level and misfortune strikes.

This is frequently the case with food allergy. A lot of patients suffer if they exceed their tolerance level for certain foods and beverages—foods and beverages they *tolerate* poorly—and *accumulate* enough to bring on illness.

Although many quick-striking food reactions are dangerous and even deadly, these aren't. Slow-acting, accumulative food reactions cause pain and discomfort but usually aren't life threatening. And unlike quick-striking food reactions, which are usually easy to diagnose, accumulative reactions require a lot of detective work. Diagnosis can be frustrating and perplexing.

When our patients eat or drink too much of a food or beverage they tolerate poorly, a number of factors can conceal the cause of illness: multiple foods are usually involved; their effects can be additive; the time of onset of illness is variable; the foods are often considered healthy; they may be disguised by food craving; symptoms are usually multiple, with many ill-defined.

Earlier we discussed the difficulty of diagnosing food allergy when many foods are involved. This difficulty is compounded with accumulation when the effects of these foods are *additive*. Eating a small amount of a number of offending foods is the same as eating a large amount of one food. For instance, if too much orange juice makes your stomach cramp, you might think you can solve the problem by drinking only one little glass a day.

It's not that easy. If you don't realize that strawberries and tomatoes reinforce the painful effects of orange juice, your tummy will continue cramping and you will continue aching, discouraged because you feel you missed the diagnosis. Don't give up; there may be a family of foods bothering your stomach. Be glad you found one of them, and look for brother and sister foods that *add* to the distressing cramping caused by orange juice. Reducing those foods will probably calm your stomach.

How soon after a meal will symptoms strike? How long does it take to fill a bucket? The answers are the same. If the bucket is empty, it may take a long time to fill it. If it is full, it may slop over if you add a single drop of water. In accumulative food allergy, it may take hours to a day or more for illness to strike—or you may not even get sick—if you haven't had aggravating foods in your diet lately. You don't have enough in your body to cause a reaction. However, if enough of these foods were featured in your recent meals, you may be like that full bucket that can't hold even a tiny bit more water. You could react quickly. That's why the time from eating to onset of symptoms is *variable*. It can range from minutes to hours to days, a variation that can be very confusing to you and your doctor.

Time of onset also varies depending on the *amount consumed*. A little bit may be okay—no symptoms. A larger amount may cause a mild reaction the next day. A meal featuring lots of an aggravating food forces early and severe discomfort. Even more variability and more confusion.

I am reminded of Jack's case of migraine headaches. Jack owned a local franchise of a major restaurant chain, so his attention was naturally directed to foods as a possible cause for his migraines. But Jack was confused. Sometimes he was sure certain foods caused the migraines; the pain struck right after he ate them. Sometimes he was sure they didn't; he ate them without experiencing pain or the headache appeared the next day. When his neurologist couldn't explain these odd circumstances, he sent Jack to see me.

The answer was obvious. Jack was affected by **multiple** foods, his symptoms appeared only after he had **accumulated** enough to have a headache, the foods were **additive** in their effects, and all of this induced **variability** in the time of onset of his headache pain.

When we identified the group of foods that caused his migraines and explained why he experienced variability in his symptoms, Jack was able to avoid food-caused migraine headaches. As long as he doesn't cheat on his diet (he does at times), food doesn't give him headaches.

Two other factors interfere with the diagnosis of food allergy. One is craving. I don't know why the sublime architect of allergy ordained that many humans (not all) must crave the foods that harm them. Maybe it was that

rascal assistant architect who burdened us with this devil-
ish perversity. I do know that it often blocks a patient from
accepting our advice on which foods to avoid.

I know the craving factor is operating when a patient
tells me, "I can't believe these foods cause me any problems." Or, "That can't be right. These foods don't bother
me." These are characteristic responses from patients with
food cravings who don't even want to consider the possibility that the foods they love are causing their discomfort.
You might wonder how we can be so sure this is a form of
denial in certain patients. The answer is simple. After they
learn these foods really are bad for them—typically about
three years later—they admit their food cravings made
them reject our advice. (I don't know why it so often takes
three years, but it does.)

The other factor interfering with the diagnosis of food
allergy is past and present training. We are **conditioned** to
believe that certain foods are healthy; we are **persuaded**
that we must eat them every day because they are essential;
we are **convinced** that without them we are unhealthy.
Mama told us, teacher told us, and now dieticians and
other health experts tell us this is true. Unfortunately for
we allergic people, mama, teacher, and these other experts
were and are mistaken, but how hard it is for us to discard
this well-meant but wrong advice.

Each of the foods and food chemicals we will discuss in
this book are defended vociferously by acknowledged
experts in food science who honestly believe they are safe
and part of a healthy diet. Many scientific studies confirm
the conclusions of these experts. Unfortunately, the allergies of my patients deny the value and safety of these foods
for many allergic patients.

This lifelong conditioning is the reason so many allergic
folks continue to consume the foods and beverages that
harm them: "After all," they tell themselves, "orange juice
has a lot of vitamin C." It's also the reason so many doctors

are unaware of the illness certain foods can cause some allergic patients: "Can't be milk. It's such an important source of calcium." And it's also the reason a patient often resists our advice: "Can't be wheat. Mother always said bread was the staff of life."

Prior and present conditioning definitely complicate the diagnosis and treatment of food allergy. So many people find it ridiculous to even suspect that the vitamin-packed glass of orange juice clutched in their fists also packs a lot of misery. Persuading them otherwise is often quite a job.

It's Not Hopeless

This lengthy discussion of the complexity of food allergy might suggest that diagnosis is hopeless, but that's not really the case. It is true that sometimes we fail to diagnose or help our food-sensitive patients, but in most cases we succeed because food allergy has one helpful trait. Each food (or group of foods) tends to cause characteristic symptoms. Not all the time, but enough times to be helpful in diagnosis. After years of diagnosing and treating food allergy, a doctor is able to recognize and use this tendency to help his patients.

Another factor that makes the diagnosis and treatment of food allergy possible is that certain foods, beverages, and food chemicals are almost always the worst offenders. They share the characteristics we already discussed: they are *multiple, accumulative, additive,* and they cause symptoms that are *variable in time of onset.* Once a patient recognizes and determines his or her *tolerance* for them, a lot of the mystery surrounding food allergy disappears. These extremely important foods and beverages are the focus of this book.

Citrus

The events that change our thinking are often peculiar. They usually leave a lasting impression because they are so strange and surprising. They challenge our deeply held beliefs, our concept of order, our most sacred convictions. They turn our view of the world upside down— and stick in our memories.

I remember just such an event, the event that forced me to develop a food allergy diet.

A Peculiar Event

It was 1965, and I was a captain in the U.S. Air Force, stationed at Offutt Air Force Base in Omaha, Nebraska. Medical school and internship completed, I was serving as a GMO (General Medical Officer) at the base hospital and clinic. There were a number of clinics, including pediatrics, internal medicine, OB-GYN, and several other specialty clinics, but there was no allergy clinic because, before I arrived on base, no doctor had been interested in this specialty. Well, I was interested. Even though I had no allergy training at that time, I realized we could improve the care of the allergic patients on base if we had a clinic that combined a doctor interested in allergy with nurses trained in allergy. I decided to start an allergy clinic.

One of my first allergy patients was five-year-old Susie, dark-haired and adorable, a little sprite with the behavior of a scamp—and skin the texture of course-grained sandpaper. She was suffering from a horrible case of eczema. Her skin was dry, thick, and red, and her constant itching and scratching made her days and nights miserable. Although this aggravating affliction didn't seem to dim her sunny disposition, I felt so sorry for her. I could see this same pity in the eyes of her father Bob, who brought her repeatedly to my clinic hoping I could help.

I tried. I prescribed all the treatments that are supposed to relieve eczema symptoms—antihistamines, salves, lotions, avoiding soap, cutting fingernails short, and wearing gloves at night to reduce damage caused by scratching. The results were frustratingly inadequate.

Then, one day Bob brought Susie in and she looked great! There had to be a seventy-five percent improvement in the condition of her skin, and she was no longer red as a lobster.

"Bob, Susie looks great." I said.

"She sure does," he replied.

"I was hoping my treatment would do Susie some good, Bob, and it looks like it finally did," I said, my head swelling with pride that I had been able to conquer Susie's severe eczema, grateful that my training and knowledge could provide such excellent results.

"Well . . . , not exactly," said Bob, with an odd look on his face.

"What do you mean, 'not exactly'?" I asked

"Well," said Bob, "none of those things helped Susie very much. She has her own way of treatment."

"Her own treatment? What is it?" I asked, wondering what it could possibly be.

"Well, when her skin gets really bad, she dumps kitchen cleanser into a bathtub full of water and jumps in. Clears her skin right up."

I was so astonished by his answer you could have knocked me over with a feather. In fact, I would have dropped if someone had waved a feather anywhere in the vicinity. Such humbling experiences are typical in my life. It seems like whenever I start thinking how smart I am, something happens to deflate my ego, letting me know I still have a lot to learn. All my fancy treatments were no match for Susie's. Move over, you gods of medical progress— Madame Curie with your x-ray machine and Alexander Fleming with your discovery of penicillin—here comes Susie with her kitchen cleanser!

Before we go any further, I want you to understand that I am not advocating your self-treatment of eczema with a bath of kitchen cleanser. I have no idea whether kitchen cleanser baths are harmful, so please don't try them.

I wasn't sure what lesson I was to learn from Susie. It was like listening to the beating of distant drums; I could sense there was a message in it for me, but I didn't know how long it would be before I could understand it. What I did know was that I wanted to help children and adults with eczema, to come up with treatments that would have better results than those available at the time provided. And I somehow knew that before I could unlock the mystery surrounding the diagnosis and treatment of eczema, I would need specialty training in allergy and the practical knowledge I would accumulate over years of treating allergic patients.

Another Peculiar Event

Before I could begin to grasp the point of Susie's lesson, however, another peculiar event occurred, one that was no less surprising than the first. Like my experience with

Susie, it made me doubt things I firmly believed to be true, made me discard tried and true methods, and shook the very foundations of everything I had been taught about allergy.

It happened years later, after I finished allergy specialty training at the Mayo Clinic and started my practice in St. Paul. It was the fall of 1973, my third year of practice, and increasing numbers of patients were visiting my office. One of these patients was a seven-year-old boy named Mike, a bright boy with the solemn manner of a supreme court judge and skin that was dry, scaly, and inflamed. In retrospect, his skin was a lot like Susie's, although it didn't occur to me at the time. If it had, perhaps I might have been prepared for the surprise that awaited me in Mike's case.

Treatment of eczema hadn't improved much since I had had Susie as a patient; results were still frustratingly inadequate. Mike had been sent to me by his dermatologist to see if I could find any causes for his rash. I wasn't too hopeful, since medical science still didn't understand eczema very well.

Mike, his mother Karen, and I tried various eczema treatments for several months without making any progress; Mike was as red and itchy as the day he first came to my office. Then, on one of Mike's visits, Karen and I had a conversation that forever changed my thinking on and treatment of eczema. I still remember that day.

"Well, Karen, how's Mike doing?" I asked.

"No change, Doctor Walsh. He's still uncomfortable and itches as much as always."

"That's too bad, Karen. I wish we could be more effective in treating him, but it's hard to do much when we don't even know the cause of eczema." Then I asked, "Karen, have you noticed anything that makes his eczema worse?"

Karen didn't take long to answer. "Yes, I have," she said. "His skin flares up whenever he eats or drinks too much citrus."

Her answer stunned me. Karen had always impressed me as being a practical and bright woman, not at all likely to be led astray by those old folk tales that blame the acids in foods for imagined illnesses. Allergy experts I respected discredited such addled-brained theories, maintaining that they were the invention of the charlatan doctor and the neurotic patient. It couldn't be true, and of that I was sure! Being relatively new to practice, I still hadn't learned to trust my patient, and I still had the inflated ego of the newly trained specialist—I fought against any new ideas that contradicted the teachings I had so laboriously pounded into my head. Thankfully, the realities of medical practice eventually deflate that ego.

Karen's belief that citrus caused Mike's eczema was contrary to everything I knew about allergy. Most allergists agree that eczema is strongly stimulated by allergy, but the idea that patients could be allergic to citrus was preposterous.

Karen's conclusion didn't make sense for a couple of reasons. First, although people who are allergic to such things as seafood or ragweed react to only tiny parts of the food or pollen, the parts must be at least a certain size. If they are too small, there is no allergic reaction. Citrus is too small. Like the toy poodle at the dog track, it doesn't belong in the race at all.

Second, most of the allergies we know about are directed against proteins; citrus isn't a protein. Most allergies are directed against proteins foreign to the body; citrus isn't foreign. In fact, *citric acid* is present in every cell in the body and is one of the compounds involved in energy production. Again, this toy poodle didn't belong in the race.

"Karen, you surprise me," I said. "I thought the fear of food acids was dead and buried. What makes you think citrus bothers Mike?"

"Because he breaks out badly if he eats oranges or grapefruit," she answered, "and he is also miserable if he drinks citrus juices or pop flavored with citrus."

I still wasn't convinced, but I put aside my skepticism for the moment and said, "Okay. Let's get citrus out of his diet and see what happens." I figured it couldn't hurt; I wasn't helping Mike much anyway.

Over the next several weeks, Karen eliminated from Mike's diet all citrus fruits, their juices, and any beverages flavored with citric acid such as pop and sports drinks. Mike's skin improved remarkably. And not only did his skin improve with citrus eliminated, returning these foods and beverages to his diet made his skin red, scaly, and itchy again. Karen was right; it was citrus—the toy poodle of allergy—that was making Mike miserable.

The results made me glad I had overcome my skepticism, and once I absorbed the implications of citrus-caused allergy, I was eager to try citrus elimination on patients with other allergic illnesses. I tried it on patients with abdominal cramps and diarrhea; the cramps diminished and the diarrhea subsided. I tried it on patients with hives; the hives were less severe. I tried it on patients with stuffed noses; the stuffiness decreased. Asthmatic patients wheezed less. Even hay fever patients responded to elimination; if they avoided citrus their pollen reactions eased up. I was impressed and excited.

Obviously citrus bothered a lot of my patients and was important in many of their allergic illnesses. But why? I can't say for sure, but I suspect it may have something to do with the human body's ability to adapt to change. Even though each one of our cells contains a small amount of citric acid, our bodies may be unable to handle large amounts of food acids. This is probably because these large quantities of acidic foods are a recent addition to our diets, and our digestive, metabolic, and elimination processes haven't yet adjusted to dealing with them.

I know this may seem surprising, since experts believe citrus cultivation started in China *four thousand years ago*. But when you consider that we digest, metabolize, and eliminate our food the same way as our primitive ancestors who dodged the footsteps of dinosaurs *eighty million years ago*, four thousand years is but a blink of evolution's eye. Not enough time to *evolve* an innovative ability to handle a *new* diet.

Our modern food production system is partly responsible for us consuming huge amounts of food acids—just check the ingredients on the canned and packaged foods in your pantry to see how many contain acidic ingredients. And our present generation's eating habits have increased the incidence of acidic foods in our diet—*grapefruit juice* in the morning, *tomato* slices in our sandwiches and an *orange* at noon, *potatoes* and *strawberry* ice cream at dinner, and *grapes* as a late-night snack.

This list emphasizes another surprising point; all of the foods mentioned are acidic. I didn't know foods such as strawberries and potatoes were acidic when Karen told me about Mike's reaction to citric acid, but I learned they were when I learned about certain inconsistencies that arose in treating other patients. Why did Dick's migraines strike when he drank apple juice, which contains mostly *malic acid*? Why did Alice's diarrhea flare up after eating candy with *fumaric acid*? Obviously, allergic distress was being caused by acids other then citric acid.

Citric, fumaric, malic acids—the names are familiar. Each of them participates in the Krebs cycle, the process that changes food to energy. As energy is released, the acids are torn apart, changing them from one acid into another. Citric acid changes to succinic acid, succinic acid to fumaric, fumaric to malic, then—after a little repair to the torn-up acid—back to citric acid again.

Of all the acids we find in our diet, citric acid is most important because it is the one most widely used. Its pleasant, sour, fruity taste makes it a perfect flavoring agent for beverages, candy, pies, and many other treats. It is often used in the pharmaceutical industry, usually in amounts too small to cause symptoms. Except in one case I remember well.

I met Jean, a seventy-six-year-old retired kindergarten teacher, when her internist asked me to examine her in the hospital just after her bowel surgery. Prior to surgery, she was given medicine to clear all the stool out of her colon. The medicine worked too well—she had a frightful case of diarrhea. Not only did she have diarrhea, she had such low blood pressure she almost went into shock, and it took days for her to recover from this overpowering reaction. Her internist and surgeon were stumped: "All we gave her was a dose of harmless magnesium citrate," they told me. *Citrate* is another name for citrus, and after battling my patient's citrus-caused diarrhea, I wasn't stumped by what happened at all, nor did I think citrate was harmless. However, the experience did help me realize that other doctors had no concept of the illness that could be caused in certain allergic patients by large doses of citrus.

Malic acid, the major acid in apples, is second in importance and frequency of use to citric acid. Much like citric acid, it has a pleasant, sour, fruity taste and is used to flavor foods and beverages and in pharmaceutical products.

Fumaric and succinic acids are seldom used in foods or beverages, although I have noticed fumaric in some candies, and both are used in drug manufacturing, where the levels seem too low to bother my patients. The names of these acids can sometimes be confusing. For all practical purposes, citrate and citric acid are the same, as are succinate and succinic acid, fumarate and fumaric acid, and malate and malic acid.

The more I investigate acidic foods and their effect on my poor patients, the more complicated it becomes. Multiple foods, multiple illnesses, multiple acids. Every time I think I finally understand it all, new information surfaces. It's like carrying a sheet of four-by-eight foot plywood on a windy day—every time you take four steps forward, a new gust comes along and blows you two steps backward.

For instance, just as I was congratulating myself on knowing all the acids that made my patients sick, I found a new one. *Tartaric acid* or tartrate, the main acid in grapes, grape juice, grape-flavored drinks, wine, and brandy, causes particularly severe reactions in my patients, illnesses such as headaches, hives, eczema, cramps, diarrhea and many others. That discovery taught me to be constantly on the lookout, and even now, although the diet works well for my patients, I am sure I haven't identified all the foods, illnesses, or acids that may cause problems. In treating food allergy, keeping an open mind is essential.

When I first began telling my patients they might be allergic to acidic foods, they were overwhelmed by the complexity of changing their eating habits, and I couldn't blame them for looking at me with evident confusion and asking, "What should I avoid?" A mumbled response that they should avoid all acidic foods didn't ease their confusion one bit. They needed to have the diet written down so they could understand it, so I began to do so. And revised it when my staff and I learned more. And revised it again and again and again. And that's how the diet has evolved to where it is today.

I believe that understanding the role of acidic foods is a significant advance in the science of medicine and the diagnosis and treatment of medical illness. But lest you think I am praising myself, let me hasten to say I didn't discover it. Susie and her kitchen cleanser baths, Karen and her theory on citrus, as well as many other patients who contributed their insights—they all helped.

By the way, I'm sure you must be wondering why it helped when Susie bathed with kitchen cleanser. I have to confess I'm not sure, but I think I know. Susie was neutralizing the acidity of her skin by soaking in bath water turned basic by kitchen cleanser. It is a basic law of chemistry that in solution, bases neutralize acids. I believe that in cases like Susie's, the body is trying to eliminate the excess acid in the diet by dumping it on the skin, where it causes the redness, scaliness, and obnoxious itching characteristic of eczema.

Perhaps Susie's kitchen cleanser is a key to learning the cause of this annoying condition.

Monosodium Glutamate (Alias MSG)

A doctor's mission and calling is to nurture, protect, and improve his patients' precious health. This honorable mission imposes a heavy burden of responsibility on members of the medical profession, an obligation to shield our patients and the community at large against what we perceive as dangerous. I believe all doctors feel this obligation. I know I do.

For me, nothing heightens this sense of obligation more than monosodium glutamate, a food chemical my staff and I try our darnedest to eliminate from our patients' diets. I don't mean to be an alarmist, but I am deeply worried by the frequency with which I encounter its effects in my practice and its presence in so much of what we eat. Perhaps when I tell you about some of my experiences with this dietary chemical, you'll understand my concern.

Citrus Wasn't Enough

I was delighted with the improvement in my patient's symptoms when the significance of the acidic foods and beverages became apparent. When patients reduced or eliminated them, headaches decreased, cramps and diarrhea slowed down, hives sprouted less often, eczema itched less, noses unblocked, and wheezing declined.

However, I was also perplexed. Although my patient's symptoms diminished, they did not disappear. In fact they still had plenty of headaches, hives, diarrhea, and all the other maladies to which the allergic person is prey. I had to improve the diet.

Fortunately, I was able to find a number of good references that helped. Through them I learned that many foods other then oranges, lemons, limes, and grapefruit are acidic. Tomatoes, berries, and cherries are acidic, often more so than the citrus fruits. And the acid in grapes—tartaric acid—can stimulate especially vicious allergic symptoms. Apparently, that's why so many of my patients can't drink wine.

That the ordinary potato is acid came as quite a shock to me. It wasn't even on my list of suspects. The potato seems to be related to the tomato; to me the leaves look like tomato leaves and the seed looks like a tiny green tomato. That helps explain why many of my patients suffer if they eat potatoes. I found that potatoes cause the same symptoms as tomatoes if eaten in excess of my patient's tolerance level, a level that is sometimes very low.

Each new finding was added to the diet, each new finding helped my patients, but I was still puzzled. Although there were pleasing improvements, my patients still had plenty of symptoms. Why? What was missing?

What was missing was my willingness to listen to my patients. I hadn't yet learned the lesson that the ones who knows the most about the cause of my patients' illnesses and the environmental factors that are affecting them are the patients themselves. They were telling me about other ingredients in the diet that made them ill, foods that were not acidic. I was finally forced into recognizing this by a friend who suffered with cluster headaches.

Another Ingredient in the Diet

Although the many allergies bestowed on me include sinus headache, I am fortunate in never having experienced cluster headaches, one of the most painful of human afflictions. In cluster headaches, the nerves of the face and scalp ache with overwhelming intensity. John had such headaches and had tried every medical treatment known. His only relief was to inhale pure oxygen when one of these painful headaches struck.

I tried treating him with allergy injections and eliminating acid from his diet. It helped, but he still had unexplained headaches. Then one day John complained of a particularly brutal headache, which prompted the following discussion.

"Bill, I had a horrible headache last night."

"How did it happen, John?" I asked.

"I was at a meeting where they served snacks," he said. "I wasn't hungry, but you know how you munch just to keep your hands busy. I ate some sausages that were excellent. On the way home I got hit with a headache so painful I had trouble seeing where I was driving. It was so bad I wasn't able to break it with oxygen," he sighed. "The pain kept me up all night."

"John, did you eat anything else?" I wondered.

"No."

"Did you drink anything?" I tried again.

"Just water," he replied, shrugging his shoulders.

I felt sorry for John. He looked pale and worn out after his night of dreadful pain. I was also curious—was there some clue to John's pain in that sausage? We tracked down the ingredients and found that they included monosodium glutamate.

I remembered that patients had often told me monosodium glutamate (also known as MSG) caused them headaches or diarrhea, but I had dismissed their observations, theorizing that it wasn't the MSG but their own imagination that was at fault. After all, studies by medical scientists showed that monosodium glutamate rarely, if ever, caused illness. But I was to find my patients observations were right.

What Is Monosodium Glutamate?

For those who aren't familiar with MSG aside from seeing it listed among those strange-sounding, synthetic chemicals on food product labels, a short description might be useful. First of all, it's not strange or unnatural; it's found in your body proteins. And it's also not synthetic. Every plant and animal manufactures it.

Proteins are made of individual amino acids, much as a chain is made of individual links. Glutamic acid is one of the amino acid links in protein, where it makes up from ten to forty percent of various proteins (that's a lot). When glutamic acid is freed from the protein chain, it is soluble (floats) in water or body fluids, where it meets a sodium molecule (part of table salt) that floats with it. Hence the name monosodium (one salt) glutamate (free glutamic acid)—shortened to MSG. (Sodium glutamate would be an adequate name, but someone must have decided monosodium glutamate sounded classier.)

How does it harm my patients? I believe the problem does not stem from the glutamic acid in protein, where it is bound firmly and released slowly, slowly enough so the body can handle it at its own pace. Free glutamic acid, MSG, is not bound to protein and is probably absorbed so fast that the body's metabolism is overwhelmed. It can't handle it. Foods and beverages with high levels of MSG make my patients sick with dependable regularity.

Illness Caused by MSG

The illness caused by MSG varies among patients. Debbie, a thirty-one-year-old labor and delivery nurse from one of our local hospitals, recently told me about her reactions.

"How are the allergy shots treating you, Debbie?"

"They help a lot as long as I get them every two weeks," she said. "If I let them go beyond two weeks, my nose gets stuffy and I feel tired."

"How about your diet? Any foods give you trouble?" I asked.

"I have to avoid the acid foods or I my cold sores flare up. As a nurse I look horrible with a big cold sore on my lips, and my patients think I have some terrible disease."

"Any trouble with MSG, Debbie?"

"I have to avoid it completely. I read every label, so it's not too hard to avoid in my own cooking, but sometimes I'll eat it at a restaurant or at dinner at a friend's house. I'm too embarrassed to ask them if they use MSG," she admitted. They'd probably think I'm a kook."

"I know what you mean about eating at a friend's house," I sympathized. "What does MSG do to you?"

"It's really bad, Doctor Walsh. First of all I develop a terrible thirst. Then I get puffy and bloated and my clothes get real tight, and I can't wear a belt because my stomach hurts. I get hyper, and for several nights I can't sleep. And all my joints ache."

Debbie's reaction to MSG is not rare, unusual, or a figment of her imagination. Many other patients complain of these symptoms, and I also share them. I always ask at a restaurant if they use MSG and try to choose foods that aren't likely to contain it, but sometimes I get it anyway. My good friends know not to use it in meals they prepare for me, but I feel strange questioning the hostess about MSG if I don't know her well. Like Debbie, I don't want to sound like a kook.

When I get MSG, it gets me. Hours later a huge thirst develops; I feel puffy and bloated—my hands swell so much they feel like sausages. My belt hurts and my bathroom scale creeps upward, showing five extra pounds that stay for about three days, then drop off. (I often wonder how many people who are taking "water pills" for fluid accumulation share this problem.) After eating foods with MSG, I sleep miserably for about three nights until the bloating stops and the scale drops. My stomach churns with acid, and like Debbie, I have nagging joint pain; my bad knee swells and aches for three days.

So for many patients MSG causes puffiness, bloating, abdominal discomfort, joint achiness, irritability, and insomnia. And the list of symptoms goes on and on. For others, their asthma worsens, their noses stuff and their ears block, hives flare, and eczema itches more. For those who react with headaches, their sinus pressure increases measurably, and migraine sufferers experience nearly unbearable surges of pain. (I don't think any of my numerous patients with frequent headaches can tolerate MSG.)

In the majority of my patients who develop pain and discomfort from MSG, although the reactions brought on by this food additive are not life-threatening, they find its effects so devastating that many must avoid it as they would avoid playing with a loaded gun.

At the same time, the subject of MSG must be approached with a sense of proportion. It does not cause all allergic symptoms, although it causes many. Allergy is too complex a matter to attribute all symptoms to a single food or food chemical; logic tells us there have to be multiple causes for these numerous illnesses. However, it is important to recognize that, in my patients, this dietary component often provokes uncomfortable, painful, and even dangerous illness. I suspect that my patients are not atypical and that many other allergic people share this susceptibility to MSG.

Where Is MSG Found?

When I began looking for acidic foods, I foolishly thought they would be easy to find. Instead, I found there were many sources and types of acids, and they could crop up in the strangest places. It was the same with MSG.

At first I thought, *What could be easier?* Read your labels, stop using spices that contain MSG, and when you dine out, tell the waitress you want your meal prepared without it. The problem is solved. Unfortunately, it's not that easy.

When you tell the waitress not to use MSG, she often looks at you with a confused expression and asks, "What's MSG?" Or, even worse, she will attempt to appease you by assuring you, "We don't use MSG in our cooking," and then unwittingly bring you a meal loaded with it. How often that's happened to me.

Reading labels is the right thing to do, but you *must read every label*. MSG is used to enhance the flavor of many dishes, especially meat, breading, and soups, but you can find it anywhere in the diet. Read every label, *always*.

MSG must be mentioned on every label where it is used in its pure form. However, if a food processor added it as hydrolyzed vegetable protein, it can be present in a food without being listed on the label. I am sure the food manufacturer means no harm by not mentioning the presence of MSG in its hydrolyzed vegetable protein. After all, MSG *is* on the FDA's "generally recognized as safe" (or GRAS) list of flavoring agents. However, for my patients, not listing MSG on the label has the same effect as if the manufacturer were doing it in a sneaky and underhanded way. It often catches them by surprise.

Hydrolyzed vegetable protein is simply vegetable protein that is hydrolyzed or broken down into amino acids. Since protein, including vegetable protein, is ten to forty percent glutamic acid, hydrolyzed vegetable protein contains between *ten and forty percent monosodium glutamate*. (Remember, protein-bound glutamic acid doesn't hurt my patients. The harm comes when the glutamic acid is released from the protein and becomes the free and rapidly absorbed monosodium glutamate.)

I once went to a food show where soup processors were proudly advertising their "MSG-free" products. When I read the label, I noticed that each soup contained hydrolyzed vegetable protein. I'm afraid I made a spectacle of myself berating the poor salespeople about their suspicious advertising practices and telling them that if my patients ate their soups, they would become exceedingly ill. I didn't make any headway, but you can make a difference if you see a product with hydrolyzed vegetable protein that is not labeled as containing MSG. Complain to the store manager—he doesn't want to lose you as a customer. When *he* complains to the food companies, perhaps they will listen and admit to using MSG in their product.

Another way to manufacture MSG is to allow yeast to digest itself and, in doing so, cause the digestive enzymes to release glutamic acid from the yeast protein, producing MSG. This product is called *autolyzed (self-digested) yeast or yeast extract.*

By the way, when dining in a restaurant, ask for a simple meat, fish, or poultry dish—no sauces—and ask that no spices of any sort be put on it. Then hope for the best.

Fermentation and MSG

I thought I had discovered all the sources of MSG when I found it in spices and in hydrolyzed vegetable protein. I was wrong. Some of my patients told me they had MSG-like symptoms when they ate cheese. That sounded strange because cheese is made of milk, and milk doesn't have high levels of MSG, but I searched and found reference books on MSG which explained the mystery. (Actually, I should have figured this one out myself.)

Milk protein is twenty percent glutamic acid, most of it firmly bound to protein so that the body can slowly digest and absorb it. However, in the cheese-making process, the milk protein is fermented, breaking apart the protein and releasing MSG. It seems that the more aged the cheese, the more milk protein is digested, and the more MSG it contains. In fact, much to my distress, as I like cheese, some of the foods highest in MSG are varieties of aged cheese. What a shame.

Any fermentation process will break down protein, releasing MSG. Soy sauce, a frequently used fermentation product, contains MSG, and my patients find they must avoid it or suffer severe consequences. Fermentation may also be one of the reason so many allergic patients can't tolerate alcoholic drinks. Most of my food-sensitive patients react severely to wine, probably because the combination of citric and tartaric acids plus the fermentation-released MSG is devastating. The moral of the story? Beware of all fermented preparations.

High Free Glutamate Levels in Certain Foods

Another discovery I have made in reading about this problem is that certain foods naturally contain high levels of free glutamic acid or MSG, and patients with sensitivity to MSG must approach them cautiously. They include peas, corn, mushrooms, and tomatoes.

Eating *peas* and *corn* may be acceptable for many MSG-sensitive people. I suspect a good boiling will remove much of the water-soluble MSG, especially in corn when it is removed from the cob before boiling. Cutting it from the cob also cuts each kernel, exposing it to the boiling water.

I have personal experience with corn intolerance. I consider corn on the cob to be one of the foods of the gods. I love its sweet, succulent taste, especially when drenched in butter, but it doesn't love me. Corn on the cob gives me all the same symptoms I get from eating MSG—bloating, acid stomach, insomnia—but corn cut from the cob and then boiled is okay. A surprising number of my patients share similar experiences.

Mushrooms and *tomatoes* cannot be processed the same way. In fact, removing the MSG from these foods would probably make them so bland we wouldn't care to have them in our diet. The combination of MSG and acid in tomatoes must be the reason they are so highly prized as flavoring in our foods. The presence of both must also be the reason my patients complain so bitterly of their effects. Watch out for peas, corn, mushrooms, and tomatoes!

A Letter from the Food and Drug Administration

I wondered how the Food and Drug Administration (FDA) regarded MSG, so I called them and asked for information. They sent me a report called the *FDA Backgrounder,* dated October 1991, and titled "Monosodium Glutamate (MSG)." The following items from this report are pertinent to our understanding of MSG.

The report reviews the use of MSG as a flavor enhancer for the past 2000 years. First used "in the form of a broth made with the types of seaweed known as sea tangle," it is manufactured today using starch and sugar fermentation and is called MSG or calcium or potassium glutamate. MSG is useful as a flavor enhancer in its free amino acid form, and "part of the flavor-enhancing effect of tomatoes, certain cheeses, and fermented or hydrolyzed protein products is due to the presence of free glutamate."

The FDA has conducted and continues to conduct extensive evaluations of the safety of MSG. "Until evaluation is complete, MSG remains on the GRAS [generally recognized as safe] list with a requirement that it must be identified as 'monosodium glutamate' on the ingredient label of any food to which it is added."

The FDA is concerned by the use of MSG in foods where the presence of this product is not noted on the label, for instance, when hydrolyzed vegetable protein is used without noting that it contains MSG. The FDA "is now planning to require that the phrase '(contains glutamate)' be added to labels as part of the common or usual name for these hydrolyzed protein products that contain significant amounts of glutamate. For example, the label would state 'hydrolyzed soy protein (contains glutamate).'"

Let's hope this happens and MSG is more clearly identified on the labels of the foods we buy. For those of us who must avoid it, this will be a tremendous help.

A Helpful List

Included in the letter from the FDA was a helpful (although according to their disclaimer not comprehensive) list that I am reproducing in its entirety:

A. The following ingredients contain glutamates (including MSG), with the percentages of glutamate content indicated in the parentheses:

> Monosodium glutamate (99 percent)
>
> Hydrolyzed vegetable protein, hydrolyzed plant protein, or protein hydrolyzate (5 to 20 percent)
>
> Autolyzed yeast extract (5 to 12 percent)
>
> Sodium or calcium caseinate (about 1 percent)
>
> Aged cheese, such as Parmesan and Roquefort (about 1 percent)

B. The following ingredients may contain glutamates (including MSG), but the amounts of glutamate content can range from very small to significant, depending on their formulations:

> Flavorings
> Natural flavorings
> Natural beef flavoring
> Natural chicken flavoring
> Natural pork flavoring

C. The following ingredients may contain glutamates (including MSG), but the amounts of glutamate content can range from very small to significant, depending on their manufacturing conditions:

> Bouillon
> Broth
> Stock
> Tomato paste
> Textured protein
> Whey protein
> Dried yeasts, Torula yeast, and yeast nutrients

A Note of Explanation

The reader may be tempted to decide that flavorings containing pure monosodium glutamate must be avoided because they contain 99 percent MSG but autolyzed yeast extract (five to twelve percent MSG) or aged cheese (one percent MSG) can be eaten with safety. This is not so. What matters is how much MSG ends up in the food. If the food manufacturer added a large amount of autolyzed yeast extract to the food, the content of yeast-derived MSG may be much higher in the food than if a small amount of pure MSG were added. For our purposes, it is enough to know that an MSG-containing flavoring was added—we must avoid it. Don't buy the food. Don't eat it.

This report also shows that only a small amount of MSG is needed to flavor food. I am amazed that such a small quantity of MSG—one percent—can cause my patients so much distress.

Overriding Concerns

The impact of MSG on my patients is enormous; it causes severe illness. Its constant presence in our diet makes it difficult to avoid, but the misery it causes my patients makes avoidance imperative. It is hard for me to believe my patients are the only allergic people affected by MSG. The odds are that many people who are not my patients are susceptible, and I am concerned that they are unaware of it. Being unaware, they have no way of knowing they should avoid this chemical.

I also worry that MSG may be causing more harm than the allergic illness I see in my practice. There is good evidence MSG is *excitotoxic*; that is, it excites and damages nerves. The implications of this excitotoxicity are profound, and we will examine them as we discuss other dietary chemicals that my patients must avoid.

This reported effect on nerves was discussed at some length by the Social Issues Committee of the Society for

Neuroscience, as reported in the January 1990 issue of *Science* magazine. They note that "excitotoxic compounds mimicking glutamate's actions have been found to occur naturally in some foods at levels high enough to cause brain damage when eaten. Excitotoxins have been linked to a diet-related spastic disease in parts of Africa and Asia, to a neurodegenerative disease on Guam, and to a shellfish poisoning incident in Canada that causes a form of memory loss resembling Alzheimer's disease.

They also point out that a buildup of glutamate in the brain may be a cause of brain damage in stroke, hypoglycemia, trauma, and seizure. Also, some researchers propose that the nerve degeneration in Parkinson's and Alzheimer's diseases may be due to "glutamate metabolism gone awry." These diseases caused by excitotoxic amino acids caused the committee members to worry about the use of MSG in the foods we eat.

The concern raised by the findings of this committee may be heightened by a study reported in May 1992 in the highly respected *New England Journal of Medicine*. The authors studied amyotrophic lateral sclerosis, a chronic disease characterized by progressive muscle weakness and wasting, and finally death. Better known as Lou Gehrig's disease, it kills one person in every thousand. They found a defect in the nerve cell's handling of glutamic acid that may allow this excitotoxic amino acid to accumulate around the nerve in high enough quantities to damage and ultimately kill it.

What does all of this mean? Perhaps, some critics would say, it is nothing more than another set of far-fetched claims by experts whose imaginations are working overtime, experts foolish enough to think a flavoring agent that is so safe it can be fed to babies could cause harm. I prefer to believe it may be one of those keys I talked about in the first chapter, one that will open the door to further research that will one day prove illnesses caused by excitotoxic amino acids similar to MSG may be far more common than we suspect today.

Finally, it may mean that those who feel sorry for my patients because they cannot eat MSG-containing foods are wrong. As they dine with their families on a meal of delicious turkey flavored with hydrolyzed vegetable protein, perhaps a discomforting thought should stray across their minds.

Low-Calorie Sweeteners

Of all the dietary chemicals we ask our patients to avoid, I have the least experience with low-calorie food and beverage sweeteners.

This is not the case with other dietary chemicals. Patients respond favorably when we advise them to eliminate MSG and really try to abstain from its use, but it is hard to escape this omnipresent chemical. It is added to many foods and spices as MSG, hydrolyzed vegetable protein, hydrolyzed plant protein, autolyzed yeast, yeast extract, and natural, beef, and other flavorings. Fermentation releases it from milk (cheese), soy (soy sauce), various grains, and grapes (alcoholic beverages). It is even present naturally in foods such as mushrooms and corn. Our patients find it almost impossible to consistently avoid the excess quantities that make them ill.

Avoiding acidic food is also hard; the sources are so numerous and acidic foods and beverages so delicious.

Because my patients happen onto MSG-laced meals or devour too much acidic food on many occasions, not a day goes by when I don't hear at least one or two stories of pain and suffering from their use. These stories keep problems caused by acidic foods and MSG fresh in my mind.

Not so with low-calorie sweeteners. They are easy to identify, and our patients seem to have an innate suspicion of them. Most patients eliminate them from their diet immediately and never return to using them. Therefore, it is harder to define the symptoms they stimulate.

My best glimpse at these symptoms comes when new patients who have been using high quantities of low-calorie sweeteners stop their use, or with those few patients who continue using them while following the rest of our dietary advice. These chemicals seems to cause the same symptoms we see with MSG—headache, bloating, irritability, difficulty in concentrating, hives, eczema, abdominal cramps, diarrhea, nasal blockage, wheezing, joint and muscle aches, plus many others—and eliminating them seems to reverse those symptoms.

Although I have less experience with low-calorie sweeteners than with other components of the diet, based on my day-to-day practice I believe they cause illnesses and I also believe my patients must avoid them. Proceeding on the assumption that this is correct, let's examine them further.

What are the Low-Calorie Sweeteners?

The two most widely used sweeteners are saccharin and aspartame. Saccharin is not frequently used by my patients; however, a number of them use aspartame, which sweetens a multitude of foods and beverages, including breakfast cereal, chewing gum, cocoa, instant iced tea, and alcoholic beverage mixes. Equal, a granulated sugar substitute, is made of aspartame. NutraSweet—aspartame again— sweetens many carbonated and noncarbonated beverages.

Aspartame is made of aspartic acid and phenylalanine, two of the twenty or so amino acids that the body uses to make protein. (We already know that MSG or glutamic acid is another of these amino acids.) Although they are bound together in the aspartame molecule, this molecule seems to break apart rapidly in digestion, releasing both amino acids and allowing rapid absorption into the body (as in the case of MSG).

The phenylalanine component of aspartame raises some concern. Phenylalanine causes brain damage in infants with a medical disorder called phenylketonuria, which affects about one in twelve thousand white and Asian babies and a lower percentage of African-American babies. Two percent of us carry one of the two genes necessary to pass this disorder to our children. Infants with phenyl-ketonuria become profoundly retarded if dietary pheny-lalanine is not rigidly limited.

Obviously those who have this disorder should be avoiding aspartame, and it seems to me that anyone who uses this chemical frequently should be asking: Will long-term dietary use of phenylalanine eventually harm even those who do not have phenylketonuria? Although this would be an interesting concept to dwell on, we won't. We are more concerned with the aspartic acid component of aspartame.

Aspartic Acid

I knew about aspartic acid, but I didn't pay much atten-tion to it until it was mentioned in some material I was reading about the glutamic acid element of MSG. I was for-tunate in finding a number of reference books on glutamic acid, as well as symposium papers and textbooks written by scientists who are studying it. I was unfortunate in not being able to thoroughly understand what they were say-ing. Most of the papers were directed at scientists who are familiar with the jargon of the field and not at the occa-sional allergist who might try to read them. (Allergists have their own jargon, but I've tried to spare you many of the incomprehensible words we use.)

Even though I did not fully comprehend those refer-ences, I understood certain facts that pointed to an explana-tion of my patients' unfortunate reactions to the dietary chemicals we ask them to avoid. Although the following is speculative, I believe it is true. I also believe you deserve to know these facts. They explain *why* these chemicals must be avoided.

Excitotoxic Amino Acids

In the reference works I studied, aspartic acid and glutamic acid (MSG) were mentioned together because their actions are similar. In the chapter on MSG, we looked at some of the evidence that indicates MSG may cause harmful illness. We also reviewed the concerns expressed by some scientists who question its safety as a flavoring agent in our diet.

Both glutamic and aspartic acids are able to excite or stimulate nerve cells of animals, including humans. In excess quantities, especially in the young animal, both are neurotoxic or poisonous to nerves. They are excitotoxic amino acids that can cause nerve degeneration. That's worrisome!

Of course, our ordinary diet does not subject us to the excessive quantity of these amino acids that caused nerve damage in the animal experiments. But what if there were a population of humans that suffered nerve degeneration from *long-term, low-dose exposure* in the diet? Perhaps the threat would be even greater if other diet chemicals, such as food acids, *potentiated* or aided in this damage. What if we called this population of people *allergic patients*?

Evidence

I know this theory probably sounds a little preposterous, but there is a great deal of evidence to support it. The following are examples of allergic illnesses in which nerve degeneration is a factor.

Cold sores, those recurring and unattractive ulcers of the lips, are caused by a virus infection of the nerves of the lips. My patients find that if they closely follow our dietary recommendations, especially if they drastically reduce their intake of acidic foods, their cold sores remain tiny and almost unnoticeable. In fact, I know this first hand because I get cold sores myself. Dietary avoidance does not cure cold sores, but it stops the spread of the lip rash. Evidently, the chemicals in foods (especially acids) further injure the virus-damaged nerve that is causing the ulcer, indicating they are neurotoxic to that nerve.

Another piece of evidence that is particularly impressive is found in eczema, the irritating skin disease that is marked by constant severe itching. Biopsies of eczema skin show badly damaged nerves. Many regard this evidence of *nerve degeneration* to be a consequence of eczema, but what if it is actually the cause? What if the skin nerves were injured by the dietary chemicals that cause my patients so much trouble, and the damaged nerves sent impulses of itchiness to the brain? What if this itching sensation caused my patients to scratch their skin so hard and so frequently that it became dry, red, swollen, and even cracked? Perhaps this is how eczema happens.

If this is so, then the treatment, of course, is to remove any neurotoxic chemicals from the diet. By now, you shouldn't be surprised when I tell you that removing acidic foods, MSG, and aspartic acid from the diet almost always reduces the itchiness, allowing my patients to improve markedly.

I could give you many more examples of allergic illnesses, including such common afflictions as headaches, asthma, and hives, that give evidence of nerve degeneration or excitation. In each case, the evidence is intriguing and, I'd like to think, persuasive. Suffice it to say that these examples support my theory that dietary chemicals, including food acids, may contribute to nerve damage.

This theory is especially significant because it is *key* to explaining a great deal about food allergy. It helps in understanding *why* certain things happen. For instance, why does food allergy affect so many areas of the body? It also helps explain *how* these food chemicals cause unrelated illnesses such as diarrhea and hives in the same patient.

Relationship Between Allergic Symptoms

It might not seem like allergic symptoms that affect different areas of the body are related, but they are. Food chemicals do not need to attack the colon and skin directly, just the nerves supplying the colon and the skin. The irritated nerves throw the colon into spasm, causing abdominal pain and diarrhea. In the skin, this same damage will fire off the motor nerves, dilating blood vessels (making the skin red) and allowing fluid to leak from these dilated vessels (causing the hive bump). The damaged sensory nerves in the dilated blood vessels send itch sensations to the brain. That's why we often see abdominal pain and diarrhea as well as red, itchy, bumpy skin as part of the same allergic reaction.

Nerve damage caused by dietary chemicals can also explain other allergic illnesses. In migraine headaches, the damaged nerves controlling the blood vessels of the head dilate these vessels, stretching the surrounding nerve fibers. These stretched nerve fibers ache with each pulse of blood flowing through the blood vessels, resulting in the throbbing pain associated with migraine headache.

In patients with asthma, irritated nerves controlling the air passages fire off signals that constrict the muscles of the airway and swell the lining. Airflow to the lungs decreases and my patient wheezes. In patients with nasal stuffiness, irritated and damaged nerves swell the lining of the nasal passages, blocking the nose.

We could continue to examine the role of nerve damage in numerous other allergic illnesses, but I think the examples discussed show how all these diverse illness can share the same cause—*nerve irritation and damage caused by neuroexcitatory and neurotoxic food chemicals.*

How Does This Damage Occur?

I do not know for sure, but it intrigues me that all these food chemicals—the various food acids, MSG, and aspartic acid—are prominent in the Krebs cycle. In this important process, acids are torn apart in steps, each step changing one acid to another while producing energy, the basic energy that "powers up" each cell in our bodies.

Energy production is an enormously complicated process requiring many separate subprocesses to make it work. In the allergic person, one or more of these subprocesses must be faulty or marginal, unable to tolerate any disruption. The sudden flooding of the digestive process by the various food acids or the exitotoxic amino acids is most likely the cause of that disruption.

How are nerves injured? Nerves have special metabolic needs that may be especially vulnerable to the flooding that occurs during the Krebs cycle. Excess accumulation of aspartic, glutamic, or food acids may be particularly injurious in the allergic patient.

Different Strokes for Different Folks

Different patients exhibit different symptoms when they eat and drink the chemicals we ask them to avoid. Some experience diarrhea, some have headaches, some get hives, while still others suffer from wheezing or stuffy noses. Why do allergic people show such variation in symptoms? I believe genetics and injury account for the difference.

In our practice, we treat many families with several allergy-prone members, and I am amazed by the similarity in symptoms within each family. In some, painful migraine headaches are common to many members. In other families, headaches are as rare as a Minnesota summer without mosquitos, but eczema affects both parents and children. Some gene or combination of genes dictates a weakness for headaches or eczema. In other words, I think these patients have a *genetic predisposition* for certain illnesses.

I am convinced that *injury* is another major reason patients' symptoms appear where they do. Many of our food-sensitive patients experience severe headache pain that begins in an area of the neck that has been injured by whiplash. Those with arthritis experience painful aching in the joints when they ignore their diet. Patients with intestinal inflammatory diseases such as chronic ulcerative colitis find that dietary chemicals stimulate their abdominal distress.

Injury caused by accident or disease often dictates where allergic illness will strike. Whiplash, arthritis, and inflammatory bowel disease are not *caused* by allergy, but they are *aggravated* by it. Allergy is a despicable bully because it is attracted to areas of injury, where it intensifies the pain and discomfort that already exist. That explains why many patients with illnesses which are not caused by allergy are so frequently helped by allergy treatment. It is the cop that chases away the bully.

Aspartic Acid in the Diet

Fortunately, aspartic acid is encountered less frequently in our diet than acidic foods and MSG. As with MSG, we are not concerned with the aspartic acid that is locked into protein. Digestion is slowed by the need to break the amino acid free of the protein, retarding the rate of absorption and allowing the body to handle the aspartic acid load at a more comfortable pace. We are only concerned about the aspartic acid in our diet that can be absorbed rapidly.

The most familiar source is the low-calorie sweetener aspartame, sold under the brand names NutraSweet and Equal. It is easy to avoid, and my patients generally abstain from its use.

Free aspartic acid is also found in unprocessed food. Grapefruit has appreciable quantities, grapefruit juice even more. Orange juice, strawberries, nectarines, plums, and prunes (especially dried prunes) also contain considerable aspartic acid. In addition, these fruits contain significant amounts of the citrus acids, making them doubly distressing for my patients.

My patients tolerate peaches, perhaps because they contain only half the citric and malic acid of oranges, but peach juice concentrates both as well as the aspartic acid of the fruit. This combination of citric and malic acid plus aspartic acid is a good illustration of why my patients have to avoid any fruit juice. Tomato juice, which concentrates the tomato's low aspartic acid content plus its high glutamic acid content, is another good illustration.

Reflections

Aspartic acid came into our lives as an unwelcome guest. It made the diet more complicated for my unfortunate patients and gave them yet another dietary chemical to avoid. However, its presence provided a key to understanding both the diet and allergic disorders. It drew attention to the role of the Krebs cycle in causing allergic illness, most likely through toxic or stimulating effects on the nerves. Allergic illness due to dietary chemicals seems to result from the harmful effect of these damaged or irritated nerves.

Refined Sugar

As I recall, I was feeling pretty content. My diet was in place. It was complicated, but it worked well. At first, my patients rebelled against the elimination of favorite foods, but later they praised the diet's effectiveness. There was still much to be learned about the components of the diet—MSG, acid foods, and aspartic acid—but that was gradually happening. All in all, I was satisfied.

But there were sour notes in my symphony of contentment. Word that I was actively treating patients for food allergy with a new diet was gradually spreading among my colleagues, and they were not impressed. To allergists, patients who complain of food allergies and doctors who claim they can treat them are about as welcome as a mass murderer at a homicide detectives' convention.

After all, current thinking was that food allergy was mysterious and almost impossible to diagnose and treat. I was claiming it could be diagnosed and treated if certain dietary chemicals were avoided. Many believed that most complaints of food allergy were the wild ravings of mentally unstable patients with overstimulated imaginations. I claimed that was untrue, that my patients were right in believing they were allergic to certain foods. Current teaching insisted that food allergy was rare and could only be diagnosed by elaborate feeding and avoidance trials. I claimed it was common and could be diagnosed using patient histories and skin tests, and treated using dietary changes.

I can't say I was ostracized by my fellow allergists, but I certainly wasn't gaining their respect and admiration. The ultimate blow to my ego came when my nurses attended a lecture for nursing staff from many of the local allergy offices. The speaker poked fun of doctors who were treating food allergy by describing a local allergist who had devised a "crazy diet for his mentally unstable patients." Although the speaker didn't mention me by name, it was obvious who he was talking about. My nurses were shocked. When they told me about the incident, it became clear that my colleagues regarded my work in food allergy as falling somewhere between incompetence and quackery.

There was also another discordant note. While avoiding MSG, acidic foods, and aspartic acid was preventing headaches, diarrhea, skin rashes, and many other allergic illnesses in my patients, it wasn't preventing them all. Some patients still experienced plenty of discomfort. In the back of my mind, I knew there must be other offending foods, but the front of my mind didn't want to deal with any more additions to the diet. The back of my mind eventually won out, and another dietary chemical made its way onto the list of things to be eliminated. But only after being forcibly brought to my attention by the same friend who forced me to recognize the harmful effects of MSG.

I remember that John and I often sat at his kitchen table settling the affairs of the world and sharing personal experiences. The subject of John's dreadful cluster headaches always came up in these discussions. I wanted desperately to help him control the pain from these headaches, a searing pain he could not stop but could only relieve by inhaling pure oxygen.

We tried treating John with allergy shots and he avoided acidic foods, low-calorie sweeteners, and MSG. John was sure these dietary chemicals precipitated his dreadful cluster headaches, but since he still had a lot of them, something else *had* to be causing them. What this "something else" was eluded us—until John found it.

A New Addition to the Diet

One night as we were sitting at the table, John said, "Bill, I think I've spotted something that causes my headaches."

"Great, John. What is it?" I asked.

"Sugar."

"Oh, come on, John." I retorted in disbelief. "Lots of really elegant studies have looked at sugar and found it doesn't cause any of the illnesses popular folklore blames it for. It's even accused of making kids hyperactive and irritable, and that theory's been shot down often enough. You've got to be wrong." (Open mouth, insert foot.)

"I don't think so, Bill. I love sugar. I could eat half a pound of candy at a sitting if someone left a bowlful nearby," he confessed. "I've been wondering if the sugar might have some bearing on my headaches, so I did a little experimenting. If I have more than two sugar cookies a day, I wake up with a cluster headache, but two or less and no headache."

"John, that's hard to believe," I said, shaking my head. "This happened more then once?"

"Yes," he assured me. "Cluster headaches each time."

Now for me, an auto accident, the end of the world, and the idea of adding another chemical to the diet were equally appealing. I wasn't looking forward to telling my patients that, in addition to giving up foods high in citric acids, MSG, and aspartic acid, they'd have to avoid sweets. I could guess what their reaction would be. I also dreaded to think what my fellow allergists would say about my putting stock in the sugar-is-bad folklore. Why me?

Then I began to remember other patients who had told me they thought their headaches, diarrhea, and hives might be due to sugar. At the time, I'd dismissed their observations and even argued against them, but now I decided I should at least consider the possibility. For the next several weeks, I listened closely to my patients for signs that sugar caused their illnesses, and surprisingly the signs were there. When I asked those patients who were using the diet but were still experiencing hives, headaches, and abdominal cramps to avoid sugar, many improved remarkably. Even more amazing, their symptoms recurred when they returned to using sugar. Another chemical joined our diet!

How Can Sugar Be Harmful?

The problem with sugar is similar to that with glutamic acid and aspartic acid. Locked in protein, these amino acids do not harm my patients. Trouble erupts when my patients eat excess quantities in a rapidly absorbed or free state such as MSG or aspartame.

In most natural foods, sugar is mainly locked in storage in the form of starch. In starch, each sugar molecule is tightly bound to other sugar molecules and cannot gain its freedom until digestion breaks the bonds holding it—a superb mechanism to delay the arrival of free sugar until the digestive process is ready for it. No overload. However, we ingenious humans learned to break these bonds using a process called *refining*, releasing the sweet-tasting sugar from the nearly tasteless starch. *Refined sugar* is rapidly absorbed, flooding the body with humongous numbers of sugar molecules and unleashing the illnesses that plague my patients.

Perhaps refining sugar is an example of human inventiveness outpacing our ability to tolerate the disastrous changes brought about by that inventiveness. Our metabolism was never programmed to deal with excess free sugar, and a few thousand years of evolution doesn't even come close to changing that programming.

How Does Refined Sugar Cause Illness?

Sugar is a basic supplier of energy for all animals, including humans. Its overwhelming importance in and impact on the Krebs cycle, the energy-producing process that takes place in every cell of our bodies, make it a good place to begin our search for the cause of illness, especially since the other food chemicals—MSG, citric acids, and aspartic acid—are also prominent in this cycle.

Just as gasoline is the basic fuel of the automotive engine, sugar is the fuel of the cell's energy-producing engine. Energy is released by the progressive breakdown of citric acid to succinic, fumaric, and malic acids. After the cycle is completed, sugar repairs the broken-down acid, allowing the energy cycle to start releasing energy again.

This breakdown, energy release, and repair process is extremely complex. It requires many discrete steps that are mediated by competent enzymes. If there is a weakness in any of these steps, for example, a shortage or poor functioning of an enzyme, harmful effects are likely to occur when the system is overloaded. (A case in point is that John's cluster headaches only occurred when he ate more sugar than he could tolerate.)

In discussing the other food chemicals, I pointed out evidence that these chemicals can damage nerves. The damaged nerves then activate the swelling, pain, and blockage that bring on rashes, asthma, diarrhea, and numerous other allergic illnesses. I believe the harm caused by excess sugar also may be due to its effect on nerves. This excess of sugar may have a disproportionate effect on the major nerve center of the body, the brain. Although other parts of the body accept protein and fat as well as sugar to satisfy their energy requirements, the brain accepts only sugar, which may make it especially susceptible to damage caused by sugar overload. We will discuss this point in more detail later.

Refined Sugar in the Diet

Although refined sugar does not hide in the diet, but announces its presence like a garishly painted clown, bear with me while I review some of the numerous places it can be found. Any deliciously sweet food or beverage contains sugar unless sweetened by one of the low-calorie sweeteners. A partial list includes cakes, pies, candies, sweet rolls, fudge, breakfast cereal, carbonated and noncarbonated beverages, jellies, jams, ketchup, salad dressings, ice cream, sweetened yogurt, sweetened juices, and many others. The reader will have no trouble adding to this list.

Reading the list of ingredients on processed foods and beverages will help you determine which foods are high in sugar. Food processors are required by law to list certain ingredients on the label, including sugar, with the ingredient making up the highest percentage listed first and the others listed in decreasing order. You will be surprised at the number of foods and beverages that list sugar as one of the first few ingredients.

Sugar's Many Names

Recognizing sugar can sometimes be difficult since it comes in many forms and travels under many different aliases. The following is a list of the most common ones:

Granulated sugar (refined white sugar in granulated form)
Powdered sugar (refined white sugar in powdered form)
Turbinado sugar (partially refined sugar)
Brown sugar (sugar containing molasses-flavored syrup)
Invert sugar (sugar processed with hot acid or enzymes)
Levulose or fructose (made from invert sugar)

Dextrose or corn sugar (made from invert sugar)
Lactose (milk sugar)
Maltose (sugar made from starch using yeast)
Corn syrup (partially refined starch from corn)
Molasses (partially refined sugar from plants)
Honey (refined plant sugar collected by bees)
Maple sugar and syrup (sugar from maple tree sap)

Symptoms of Sugar Intolerance

The food chemicals that bother my patients act like a gang of thieves. Each thief, by himself, might hold up a convenience store or gas station, but as a gang they might coordinate their activities to pull off the crime of the century. By working together in the gang, with each one contributing his own bit of skullduggery, they are far more powerful and destructive.

Food chemicals behave in much the same way. While my patients might have a moderate reaction to a single chemical, it is interesting to note that their symptoms are always more severe when they eat a meal high in several chemicals. The chemicals seem to *potentiate* or strengthen each others' adverse effects. Whether it is hives, wheezing, diarrhea, headaches, or another of the host of illnesses that prey on allergic people, the symptoms are far more powerful, uncomfortable, and painful.

Excess sugar affects my patients in much the same way an excess of MSG, aspartic acid, or acidic foods does. They all cause similar symptoms. In addition, like the gang of thieves where each member specializes in performing a particular crime, each of these chemicals seems to predominate in causing a particular symptom or set of symptoms.

I am extremely familiar with MSG's ability to precipitate bloating and brutal headaches (sugar also causes both, i.e., the cluster headaches John endured). I am also impressed by the ability of citric acid and its fellow acids to

provoke the itching of hives and eczema (sugar also participates). Sugar seems to have a particularly strong impact on
the nerve center of the body—the brain.

Hyperactivity and Sugar

Hyperactivity is a distressingly common and disabling
affliction. In our modern world, where education is so
highly prized, hyperactivity is a dreadful curse that
impedes the ability to learn. The hyperactive child cannot
sit still long enough to be taught, cannot remain quiet long
enough to study. Saddest of all, he or she cannot sit still
long enough for a loving parent to cuddle. Hyperactivity is
a crippling handicap.

Although most of us are aware that hyperactivity affects
many children, few realize that some adults are similarly
victimized. Like children, they are unable to remain calm
long enough to complete complex tasks or to enjoy mean-
ingful human interactions.

My patients expose me to numerous examples of food-
induced hyperactivity. A good illustration is Mary's family
of two lively little girls. By the time I walked into the examining room for our first consultation, they had partially
demolished it. Tammie was on top of the examining table,
tearing the paper to shreds, and Tracie was trying to haul
the foot stool out the door in spite of Mary's desperate
attempts to keep her from doing so.

I see hyperactivity so frequently I can spot it in an
instant. A sure sign is a child scampering around the room
like a squirrel in a cage. It's usually reinforced by a second
sign, the look on mother's face that tells me she is sorry for
the disturbance but is powerless to stop it. She *is* powerless.
You can only spank a child you love so many times before
you cannot force yourself to do it again—especially when
deep down you feel the child cannot help his or her behavior. I am one of those who believes the fault does not lie
with the child (nor does it lie with the parent).

Mary's primary doctor sent the girls to see me because of their eczema. After testing them, we discussed the eczema, and I also raised the subject of their hyperactivity, although Mary seemed hesitant to discuss it. Like many parents of hyperactive children, she seemed to have given up hope that anything could be done about it.

We discussed dietary changes, and I stressed reduction of both acid foods (to help the eczema) and refined sugar (to see if it would have any affect on the hyperactivity). When Mary and the girls returned in three months to review their progress, she was far more willing to talk. And my office wasn't demolished.

"How did the girls like the diet, Mary?"

"Not at all, Doctor Walsh. In fact, they hate it," she admitted.

"That's not strange, Mary. Lots of our patients complain about having to avoid the foods they love. Does it help the girls?" I asked.

"It's very helpful. As long as we stick to it, their skin is almost clear."

Then she told me that the only time they had broken away from the diet was at a birthday party at school. Pop, cake, and ice cream were served, and both little girls stuffed themselves.

"Next day both were full of hives and broke out in eczema," she reported. "I was surprised at the lesson it taught them, though. Neither of them will eat acidy foods now."

I wasn't surprised. Even two- and three-year-old children will avoid sweet-tasting treats if they connect them with discomfort and pain. That's why I instruct parents not to force children to follow our diet; if the diet works and the link between food and illness is pointed out to the child, he or she will avoid the offending foods. In fact, I am often astonished by the children who intuitively avoid eating or drinking foods high in illness-producing chemicals, a habit that begins long before I first see them. If "Johnny, drink your juice" provokes a mother-child battle, there's a good possibility that Johnny and juice don't mix well.

"What about sugar, Mary?" I asked.

"That part really surprised me, Doctor Walsh. Tammie and Tracie are both much calmer on the diet. Even my mother-in-law notices, and the girls' teacher is delighted."

She told me that after the birthday party, things were pretty bad. For the next two days, the girls were unmanageable, jumping from one thing to another without stopping and driving their teacher wild. The same thing happened when Mary's father-in-law brought candy to the house.

"They got into it when we weren't watching," she said. "Now there are no more sweets at home, and their teacher watches sweets in the classroom."

The only exception I make to the "let the children manage their own diet" rule is hyperactivity. Children are often unaware of their hyperactivity, so they can't see the link between it and the diet. Patients must be aware of this cause-and-effect relationship or they won't follow the diet.

"Did you try the diet yourself, Mary?" I wondered.

"Yes, I did," she said. "As a child I was hyperactive, and now I often have days when I'm tired and irritable and can't seem to think straight. (My patients refer to this as being 'spacy' or 'spaced out'.) Now, I know I'll have days like that if I eat too much sugar. I wish someone had known about sugar and hyperactivity when I was young."

I do too. I feel sorry for the many children—and adults—who never have a chance at scholastic achievement or many of life's other rewards because of their hyperactivity. Even love and cuddling are almost impossible for children who cannot sit still long enough to be held. I firmly believe their unmanageable behavior springs not from an innate and hateful defiance, but from the hyperstimulation of the various food chemicals—especially sugar.

Mary told me she was delighted with the diet's effect on her own symptoms, but she also said it was hard for her to give up sugar. She has a genuine craving for it. In fact, when she took it out of her diet, she was miserable for five days. "I felt tired and irritable, I couldn't sleep, my hands shook, and I had a horrible headache."

Sugar Craving

Mary's experience when she eliminated sugar from her diet, what in reality were nearly intolerable withdrawal symptoms, is shared by many other patients. About one out of four or five patients crave sugar; they suffer dreadfully when they eliminate it. Their symptoms vary and may include shaky hands, muscle aches and pains, perspiration, sleeplessness, striking irritability; in other words, they feel terrible.

These withdrawal symptoms form a substantial barrier to treating patients who crave sugar. It is hard for them to recognize that sugar avoidance, which brings such pain, is necessary to control the headaches, body aches and pains, diarrhea, and other distresses that brought them to my office. When a patient craves sugar enough to suffer unpleasant withdrawal symptoms when it is eliminated, *denial* often comes into play. He or she will deny even the possibility that sugar could be causing symptoms.

It is, though. Hundreds of my patients find excess sugar causes a stuffy nose or headache; hardly a day goes by when patients fail to mention the ill effects of too many treats. My staff and I have found that any food craving is a signpost pointing to the food that is almost certainly a major cause of our patient's problems. We try to identify food cravings so we can emphasize avoiding those foods or food chemicals.

I mention food craving because we encounter it so frequently and it is so difficult to counter. In many cases, patients fight this diagnosis for years and continue to suffer until they accept it. For some odd reason, it typically takes three years for the resistant patient to come around.

A good example is Judy, a thirty-five-year-old emergency room nurse I have been treating for migraines for several years. At the outset, she tried to eliminate refined sugar, suffered overwhelming withdrawal headaches and irritability, and decided sugar was not to blame. After three years, on one of her regular follow-up visits, I asked: "How are you doing, Judy?"

"Really well, Doctor Walsh. My migraines are fine as long as I get my shots every two weeks."

"What about your diet? I asked. "Do any foods bring on the headaches?"

"I have to avoid tomatoes, oranges, and MSG entirely or I get bad headaches," she said. "I also have to watch potatoes and cheese, and I can only have pizza if I don't eat any bad food for two days before the pizza."

When I asked, "What about sugar?" I was surprised at Judy's answer.

"I've eliminated it from my diet altogether. Once I start to eat sugar, I can't stop and I end up irritable, I can't think clearly, and get hit with a horrible headache."

You do not make friends when you say "I told you so," so I didn't. But I remembered three years back when Judy said the diet was stupid and sugar didn't bother her. Eventually she became convinced sugar was the culprit, but she suffered a long time before recognizing it. Perhaps her story will help others with sugar craving realize their problem.

A Reflection

I often reflect on my experiences with sugar. I was reluctant to add it to the elimination diet because it would be yet another chemical that my patients must avoid. However, together my patients and I learned it must be eliminated to truly control their distressing symptoms. Sugar's effects on the brain—sugar craving, hyperactivity, 'spacy thinking'— also forced me to confront the effect of all allergies, especially the food chemical allergies, on the central nervous system. It is this connection that ensures its permanent place in the diet.

Other Foods and Beverages

In our discussion of foods and beverages that cause my patients' reactions, I touched only lightly on several that merit further consideration. In addition, there are a few others that ought to be discussed. These foods and beverages are major components of our diet, and sensitive patients must be extremely cautious when consuming them. We will examine them more thoroughly in this chapter, as well as addressing some issues frequently raised by patients for whom I prescribe the elimination diet.

Corn

Corn deserves special attention because it is so prevalent in our modern diet and also because it is often a major problem. For many of our patients, corn provokes the same symptoms as the dietary chemicals—sugar, acidic foods, MSG, and aspartic acid. This is somewhat of an enigma because when these patients are skin tested to corn, the test is negative. This indicates that the protein in corn is not to blame (allergy to protein is the usual cause of a positive skin test), but that the reaction is more likely amino acid related.

Today's corn plant was hybridized from an American weed used for food thousands of years ago. This evolution changed it from an ear the size of a strawberry to the seed-bearing hulk grown on modern farms today. As each generation of seed was selected for its increased size, it must also have been cultivated for taste. We know that MSG gives both natural and processed foods a robust and pleasant taste, and corn is naturally rich in this free amino acid. Regrettably, the high MSG content that accounts for the pleasant taste sought by our ancestors is probably also responsible for the unpleasant reactions my patients suffer.

The ramifications of corn allergy are disturbing. Corn, which is the world's most widely distributed food crop, is found in countless products, including breakfast cereals, corn meal, many varieties of canned corn, corn bread, corn on the cob, corn starch, corn syrup, crackers, popcorn, tortillas and numerous others. Obviously, eliminating corn from the diet poses a terrible hardship. A frequent question my patients ask is whether they most avoid all corn products.

While I can't be entirely sure, I don't think so. MSG decomposes at 250 degrees Fahrenheit, and any product processed at a higher temperature presumably will be low in intact MSG. Therefore, unless MSG is added after baking, cereals, crackers, breads, and similar products are probably acceptable for patients who are allergic to chemicals.

Unfortunately, the temperature of boiling water is only 212 degrees Fahrenheit, so foods prepared in this way generally cannot be expected to be free of MSG. This must be the reason so many of my patients find that corn on the cob causes them grief. The anticipation with which we await the late summer harvest of delicious sweet corn, and the widespread popularity of this grain product, combine to obscure its obnoxious effects on my patients. They are often unaware that they are allergic to corn until we warn them to watch for symptoms after they eat it.

I share my patients' love of corn on the cob and their distress after eating it. In fact, the bloating and abdominal pains I was beset with after a delicious meal of corn on the cob first brought this food allergy to my attention.

Unfortunately, the potential for corn on the cob to cause suffering is shared by popcorn. I suspect that even the relatively high temperature required to pop corn is not sufficient to destroy the high levels of MSG.

If corn is cut from the cob and then boiled, my patients often seem able to tolerate it. With this preparation method, each of the corn seeds is cut open, which apparently allows the MSG to be dissolved and dissipated into the boiling water. Another way to reduce MSG in foods is to store them for at least twenty-four hours before preparation; stored foods contain less MSG then fresh foods.

Peanuts

I feel terrible when I tell my patients they should avoid popcorn because it often brings on reactions such as headaches, diarrhea, rashes, and the myriad other illnesses that plague the susceptible allergic patient. I feel even worse telling them that peanuts can cause the same distressing symptoms.

I know that many patients would more readily accept the need to avoid popcorn if they could substitute a crunchy handful of peanuts as they watch a ball game or snack at a party. Unfortunately for many patients, this substitution brings regrettable symptoms.

My staff and I learned about the potential for peanuts to cause harm from patients who gave up popcorn when they found it caused them to feel sick. Many of them told us that when they replaced popcorn with peanuts, they experienced the same discomfort. I know that I suffer uncomfortble symptoms from both foods.

It is surprising that pain and discomfort can be caused by such an important food source. Like corn, peanuts are a major food crop; seventeen million metric tons are grown per year and processed as peanut butter or simply roasted and sold at sporting events, circuses, etc., and as at-home snacks. Also like corn, the peanut has long been used as a human food. It is known to have existed as early as 950 B.C. in South America, and its use was widespread throughout Mexico and South America when early explorers reached these areas in the sixteenth century.

The peanut may be similar to corn in another way. Although I was unable to determine the exact MSG content of the peanut from my reference materials, I suspect that as a member of the pea family (hence the name *pea*nut), it is likely to be high in MSG. In fact, peas contain more MSG than corn. Since most of my patients tolerate boiled peas, this process must reduce the level of MSG, but unfortunately, the processing of shelled and unshelled peanuts does not seem to have similar benefits.

Oddly enough, many of my patients who cannot eat a handful of peanuts do seem to tolerate peanut butter. Perhaps the process for making peanut butter takes place at temperatures high enough to destroy MSG. We tell our patients to try eating peanut butter if they miss it in their diet; they can continue to use it as long as it does not stimulate symptoms.

A word of caution: *People who experience life-threatening symptoms (i.e., breathing difficulty, hives, loss of consciousness, or other severe reactions) from eating peanuts should never try to eat this food in any form.*

Beans can cause distressing symptoms in the allergic person, and I have personal experience with some of them. Every once in a while I have a meal with green beans or other bean products that have not been thoroughly boiled. They have a somewhat crunchy texture, and this clue to their less than completely cooked nature saves me much pain if I heed it. If I eat them anyway, I experience an MSG-type reaction (my bad knee swells, my stomach burns, and I sleep poorly at night). A good, hard boiling until the beans are soft—even mushy—spares me all this trouble. It may also spare you.

Alcoholic Beverages

Another issue our patients want to know about is consumption of alcoholic beverages. Unfortunately, because distillers and wine producers are not required to provide any information on liquor labels other than alcohol content, my advice about alcoholic beverages is based on meager data. However, certain facts can serve as a partial guide to their use.

As mentioned earlier, because fermentation of any food or beverage releases MSG as the protein breaks down, you can expect to find MSG in any alcoholic beverage. My primary advice is to drink in moderation so that you do not accumulate an excess of MSG.

Some alcoholic beverages seem worse than others. Corn-based liquors such as bourbon cause my patients great distress; they seem to tolerate grain-based beverages such as scotch much better. The same is true for beer. American beer is often brewed from corn and seems to be poorly tolerated by my patients compared to barley-based beers such as the German ales and lagers.

I also caution my patients to avoid using any mix other then water; these products usually contain high amounts of sugar and acid.

Another piece of advice I give my patients is to be extremely careful of brandy and wines, especially the red wines. Because brandy and wine are fermented from grapes and are high in both citric and tartaric acid as well as MSG, they are particularly bothersome to my patients. I recommend asking for a glass of water instead.

Yogurt

Yogurt is produced from milk by fermenting it with two bacteria. Unfortunately, this fermentation probably releases the glutamic and aspartic acids that are bound to the milk's protein, and both of these acids are irritating to my patients. The amount of these free amino acids probably varies depending on the fermentation process, as is the case with cheese; the more fermented (aged) the cheese, the more elevated the MSG content. Lacking information on the free amino acid content of various yogurt brands, it is impossible to tell which may be lowest in these acids and thus best for my patients.

Since I do not believe yogurt contains particularly high levels of aspartic acid and MSG that is free or not bound to protein, I believe most of my patients can tolerate a limited amount in their diet; however, eating a lot of it would be a great mistake. It would also be inadvisable to eat flavored yogurts, especially those that contain aspartame or citrus; the effect of the sugar and acid content combined with MSG and aspartic acid could lead to uncomfortable symptoms.

The Cabbage Family

I am surprised by the number of my patients who are sensitive to cabbage, cauliflower, broccoli, and brussels sprouts. My nursing staff and I took an informal survey and found that the majority of our patients suffer symptoms from either corn or the cabbage family. Interestingly enough, most patients reacted to one or the other, but not to both. I have no idea why this is so, nor do I know why so many react to the cabbage family. Watch for this allergy. Boiling these foods well may allow you to eat them if you react to them when they are uncooked.

Caffeinated Beverages

I am often asked by patients whether caffeinated beverages such as coffee can give rise to the some of the symptoms they experience. I am hesitant to say yes or no—mostly because I don't know.

Skin tests are a great help in diagnosing the cause of allergic disorders; they point to these causes like a signpost points out the correct road to a city. Unfortunately, because there is no skin test for caffeine, there is no signpost telling me if caffeine is a problem for my patients.

A traveler on a road with no signposts has to rely on a best guess as to which direction to take. Similarly, I have to rely on guesswork to try to answer this question. However, sometimes an event occurs that leaves such a strong impression, it influences the direction this guesswork takes.

I had such an experience while visiting a dear friend in the hospital where he was recovering from hip replacement surgery. Al and I attended medical school together, and he is now practicing in town. In the course of our conversation, he asked me if any of my patients had reported unusual symptoms associated with coffee. After confessing that I was unsure of the role of coffee in causing allergic symptoms, I asked him what prompted the question, and our conversation went something like this.

"Well, Bill, a weird thing happened to me recently," he began, with a satisfied look on his face. Al loves to tell stories, tells them well, and often makes me envious of his ability to bring a story to life.

"Tell me about it, Al," I said, curious to find out what he might have to tell me about coffee.

"Peculiar things have been happening with my vision lately," he said. "Spots float in and out, flashes of light come and go, and sometimes part of my vision is hazy and I can't see very well. I keep thinking I've got something in my eye and try to brush it away. It's really upsetting and probably dangerous, especially when I'm driving at night."

My recounting of this experience doesn't do justice to Al's ability to weave a good story about his experiences, but it does indicate the tendency for caffeine—in coffee—to cause symptoms. His symptoms were those of the aura (vision disturbance) that often precedes a migraine headache. Luckily for Al, the headache did not follow the aura, as it does in so many unfortunate people who suffer migraine's throbbing pain. But he was perceptive enough to realize his symptoms probably represented a migraine aura and to check his theory by avoiding coffee. The vision disturbances disappeared. His suspicions were confirmed by a neurologist during a "curbstone consult." (That's when a doctor calls another doctor for personal advice without seeing him in his office. Like their patients, doctors go to great lengths to treat themselves instead of seeing another doctor.)

As you can imagine, this experience makes me very suspicious of caffeine. Although Al's aura never grew to a rip-roaring headache, I see no reason it wouldn't in those who are more susceptible to this cruel pain. My suspicions are further increased because caffeine affects me. It causes abdominal cramps and burning if I take it. I must avoid caffeine.

My advice is, if you react to foods, be very careful of caffeine.

Food Supplements

Many food supplements are marketed for people on diets or for those who want to improve their strength and endurance for sports and exercise. These worry me. Many are derived from proteins that are hydrolyzed (broken down) into their constituent amino acids. This frees both aspartic and glutamic acids, and we have already discussed the effects of these amino acids. I ask my patients to avoid these supplements.

Vitamins

The question my patients ask most frequently is: "If I cut out all these foods, where do I get my vitamins?" The fact is that when you examine the foods that are acceptable on the diet, the answer is obvious. The many fresh fruits, vegetables, and meats that are allowed contain all the vitamins you need for proper nutrition. And conversely, many of the foods we recommend eliminating are not high in nutritional value.

Many people supplement their diet with extra vitamins, in most cases, the one-a-day type. For most of my patients, this is unwise; supplemental vitamins often make them ill. I confess to doing this from time to time, but a week of taking vitamins makes me so sick I am cured of the temptation.

I am not sure why vitamin supplements cause so much discomfort. One possible explanation is that they usually contain citric acid. Pharmacists tell me that vitamin C needs to be combined with citric acid to prevent deterioration and inactivation, but this is only a partial answer.

Many of my patients also react poorly to vitamins that do not contain vitamin C. In some cases, I believe this happens because they contain yeast as a source of some of the vitamins. It is not difficult to conclude that those who are allergic to yeast would develop pain and discomfort from eating it.

The fact that so many of my patients suffer bloating, diarrhea, rashes, abdominal pain, and a number of other symptoms from taking vitamins makes me wonder whether we should reexamine the value of these dietary supplements. They may not be as harmless as we think. It's like the owner of a Volkswagen "Beetle" who isn't satisfied with its ruggedness and reliability, but also wants it to accelerate like a dragster, so he drives it to the airport and fills the tank with jet engine fuel. Much to his chagrin, he finds that instead of accelerating better, the car barely operates at all because it was never designed to run on jet fuel.

Maybe vitamins are like jet fuel for our bodies. Instead of improving its operation, do they pose a threat we aren't even aware of?

Salt

Strictly speaking, salt is not a food; it is a seasoning. However, no book about food allergy would be complete without mentioning the effect of salt on patients with allergy because many of them notice excess salt increases their allergic symptoms.

How does salt cause increased symptoms for my patients? In certain people, salt seems to promote fluid accumulation, and this may aggravate the bloating effect of food reactions—a consequence my patients and I experience when our diets are too heavily loaded with foods and beverages we tolerate poorly.

If excess salt is a source of discomfort for you, it would be wise to limit your intake of salty foods.

Illnesses Caused by Food Allergy

Describing the illnesses caused by food allergy is like trying to gift-wrap an elephant—there's not enough paper to do it. What's more, even if you had enough paper, where would you start?

Now I know this analogy is a little ridiculous, but it does give you some idea of the dilemma I faced in writing this chapter. Food allergy provokes so many illnesses that to include an elaborate scientific description of all of them would have made this book so expensive the average person couldn't afford it. Besides that, I did not write this book to help you diagnose your own illnesses. Diagnosing and treating illnesses should be left to your doctor, and you should not rely on any book to diagnose yourself. Your doctor is trained to recognize symptoms and determine their cause. Go to him for help so you can avoid the mistakes that will surely result from self-diagnosis and treatment.

Instead, the purpose of this book is simply to make you more conscious of food allergy and the many illnesses associated with it. The summary of allergic illnesses in this chapter is intended to increase your awareness of their symptoms. If you are experiencing any of these symptoms, you should at least consider the possibility that they are food-related.

One way to comprehend the multitude of these ailments is to consider how food allergy causes harm. I believe allergenic foods, especially food chemicals, disrupt the Krebs cycle, the basic energy-producing sequence that supplies all the cells of the body—all the muscles, bones, skin, blood vessels, and other organs that are so essential to life. Any disruption of this process will have widespread consequences.

The Krebs cycle also energizes our nerves. Earlier I presented evidence that the discomfort and pain of allergic illness results from damage to the nerves, damage caused by an overload of the chemicals involved in the production of nerve energy. Nerves stimulate and control virtually every area of the body, so by damaging nerves, food allergy can wreak havoc anywhere in the body. It uses nerves as pathways to various parts of the body, just as we use highways to travel from one place to another. That's why my patients suffer multiple symptoms simultaneously, symptoms that make food allergy difficult to pin down because they seem to be unconnected. However, they are related through the body's intricate network of nerves.

The long list of disorders for which food allergy is the *direct cause* is augmented by numerous illnesses for which it is *indirectly responsible*. Like an inconsiderate bully, allergy seems delighted by the opportunity to further torment my patients who have non-allergy-related disease. For instance, we often see patients with back pain due to degenerated vertebrae or whiplash injury that is greatly intensified by food allergy. For patients with intestinal inflammations such as ulcerative colitis, allergy makes their bouts of painful diarrhea much more severe. In these instances, the disorder is not directly caused by food allergy, but the *pre-existing condition is aggravated* by it.

In the following summary of allergic illnesses, I won't make a point of telling you which are direct and which are indirect. Since doctors are unsure of the cause of many illnesses, it isn't important to make that distinction. The important thing is that if exposure to certain food chemicals is causing discomfort and pain, those chemicals must be avoided.

Allergic Illnesses—The Blood Vessels

The blood vessels are an appropriate place to begin our exploration of the illnesses brought on by food allergy. So many allergic symptoms can be explained in part or altogether by swelling or spasm of the blood vessels.

MIGRAINE HEADACHE. A popular theory for what causes **migraine** is that it is related to spasms of the blood vessels in the head. The resulting restriction of blood flow denies blood-borne nutrition and oxygen to the brain and eyes. This decrease in energy and oxygen produces the vision changes and numbness that warn many patients they are about to be socked with migraine's agonizing pain.

The pain occurs when the blood vessels relax because they are tired of being in spasm. Unfortunately, they relax too much and swell like a boiling sausage; the pulsating blood flowing through them stretches pain fibers, and a throbbing headache ensues.

HIVES AND ANGIOEDEMA. Anther disorder that can be explained by blood vessel changes is **hives**, a condition characterized by intensely itchy red blotches—some large, some small—caused by the swelling of small blood vessels at the surface of the skin. The swollen vessels leak fluid into the surrounding skin, causing the hives to break out. The discomfort that accompanies the hives results from irritation of the itch-sensitive nerves at the skin's surface. Not only are hives uncomfortable, they can be terribly embarrassing. Imagine going to work with red splotches all over your face!

Angioedema is a condition in which the hives form deep in the skin. Patients develop swelling that can turn fingers into sausages, raise flat-topped welts on the skin, or puff up the eyelids, hands, and feet. These deep-seated swellings, which are sometimes redder and sometimes paler than the surrounding skin, typically do not itch because the nerve fibers at the surface of the skin are not stimulated to send out an itch sensation. Often hives and angioedema strike together, and my patients suffer both the red, itchy hives and the uncomfortable swelling.

ASTHMA. Blood vessel changes can also explain some characteristics of **asthma**, which causes difficulty in clearing air from the lungs. During severe asthma attacks, the chests of victims become distended because their breath is trapped in their lungs like the air in an overinflated balloon. Exhaling, which is second nature to those without asthma, becomes an exhausting struggle.

Breathing is difficult because the passages that carry air to the far reaches of the lungs are obstructed. The blood vessels swell and leak fluid into the airway lining, much as they do in hives and angioedema. The swollen linings partially block the passage of air, producing the frightening whistle or wheezing sound that is so familiar in asthma sufferers.

The same swelling that causes hives, asthma, and migraine headaches can occur in a number of other areas. Next we'll examine the consequences of this reaction in the respiratory tract, the sinuses, the chest cavity, and the joints.

SWELLING IN THE RESPIRATORY TRACT. If the swelling centers in the vocal cords, it can cause **hoarseness and loss of voice**. This is a frequent complaint of many of my patients, especially singers, ministers, and others who frequently address the public. Perhaps the strain these activities put on their vocal cords weakens the area and makes it more susceptible to the voice changes caused by allergy.

Swelling in this same area, especially when accompanied by an annoying itch, can lead to the **chronic cough** and **persistent throat clearing** that exasperates so many of my patients. The spring and fall rainy seasons send a constant stream of coughing and throat-clearing patients to my office, usually at the request of parents, spouses, or friends who are tired of listening to this irritating noise day and night.

For a sizable share of the population, the airway swelling is so pronounced that they can actually strangle! They experience an **obstruction of the airway**—a swelling that makes it extremely difficult for them to breathe. Fortunately the strangling has not been fatal in any of my patients because the swelling has caused only a partial blockage. Needless to say, they live in fear that one of these attacks will be their last.

This frightening disorder is often misdiagnosed as hyperventilation by doctors who are unaware of this surprisingly frequent allergic reaction. Patients who suffer from angioedema in the airway usually know that something is blocking their breathing, and will even point to the spot on the neck or chest where they feel the obstruction. Their struggle for air is similar to the **hyperventilation** that accompanies anxiety attacks, but in these cases, the anxiety is brought on by the condition instead being the cause of it. Forget the tranquilizers!

When angioedema occurs higher in the respiratory tract, its symptoms are relatively harmless but unpleasant. If the swelling is at the back of the throat, it can cause recurrent **sore throats**. Although painful to my patients, these sore throats seem to have no infectious basis because they produce negative throat cultures. It can also produce **swelling of the tongue, lips, or membranes in the mouth**, as well as the most common complaint of allergy patients—**nasal stuffiness**. This unpleasant symptom, which results from swelling in the mucous membranes of the nose, is like having a constant cold with its accompanying tiredness, irritability, and just plain yuckiness. It is very frustrating to treat this condition if the patient refuses to limit the foods and beverages that promote the stuffiness.

SINUS HEADACHE. If the swelling is even higher in the respiratory tract—in the sinuses—my patients experience the nagging, steady pressure and pain of **sinus headache**. Over half of the patients who come to us for treatment have aggravating pain in the forehead, eyes, cheeks, or back of the head that is characteristic of these distressing headaches. I know firsthand how distressful they can be since I used to suffer dreadful sinus headaches. The opportunity to help others avoid these headaches is one of the things that attracted me to the field of allergy.

SWELLING IN THE CHEST. Another surprisingly common allergic symptom is **chest pain**. My patients often complain of a painful tightening or heavy sensation under the sternum (breastbone), much like that experienced by people who are having heart attacks. I imagine more than a few doctors have been surprised to have an allergic patient with severe chest pain produce a normal EKG.

SWELLING IN THE JOINTS. Since allergy is known to be a tormentor of weak or damaged areas, it is no surprise that angioedema frequently attacks the muscles and joints of patients with non-allergy-related diseases such as **rheumatoid arthritis** or **osteoarthritis**. The swelling generally occurs deep in the affected joints and is barely noticeable on the surface of the skin, producing little or no heat or redness (heat and redness are the hallmarks of arthritic inflammation). Many of my patients with arthritis experience episodes of pain in their arthritic joints when they do not watch their diet.

This same annoying pain bothers joints that have been damaged by injury. Patients with **whiplash** and other spine injury are vulnerable, as well as those with **TMJ** or **post-**

traumatic joint injury (for example, joints damaged by football injury). Here again I speak from personal experience. My "football" knee aches and swells with fluid when I exceed my tolerance for food chemicals—in my case, almost always MSG blundered into by mistake.

NERVES, BLOOD VESSELS, AND MYSTERY. Much of the mystery surrounding allergies seems to stem from the fact that they strike such widely separated areas of the body, areas as unrelated as the joints and respiratory tract. But in the previous discussion, we used a *key bit of information* to dispel this mystery.

We saw how widely separated and unrelated parts of the body are affected by the same process—swelling and spasm of blood vessels. In tracking this swelling as it moved around the body, we learned why different allergic disorders bring discomfort and pain. We also saw that areas already weakened by injury or disease as well as genetically predisposed areas can be vulnerable to allergy attack.

Now that we know allergy is not really mysterious, let's explore the relationship between the blood vessels and nerves that have been damaged by the overload of dietary chemicals.

THE RELATIONSHIP. Blood vessels can no more dilate or spasm by themselves than a car can drive itself. Imagine picking up the morning paper and reading:

MR. JONES'S 1990 HUPMOBILE JAILED AFTER BEING CONVICTED OF SMASHING INTO STOP SIGN

Upon reading this, whoever is in charge would probably make reservations for the reporter, the judge, and the arresting officer on the nearest psychiatric ward and order a trial for Mr. Jones, the car's driver.

Just as cars do not drive themselves, blood vessels do not order themselves to dilate. Nerves do, and understanding this relationship is key to understanding the effects of allergic reactions on the nerves and blood vessels.

In an earlier discussion, I presented evidence that nerves are damaged by allergy and that these damaged nerves may stimulate blood vessels to swell and leak. However, I did not mention that in addition to nerve damage, there is another mechanism that may stimulate the vessel-swelling commands of nerves.

Many of the nerves in the blood vessels are stimulated by *neurotransmitters* (chemicals that transmit or carry messages to nerves). Both MSG and the aspartic acid in low-calorie sweeteners are known neurotransmitters; in fact, they are also neurostimulating and neurotoxic (damaging to nerves). I think it is logical to assume that sugar and acidic foods are likewise damaging to nerves because they cause the same illnesses in my patients. It is possible—even probable—that the rapid absorption of these chemicals leads to blood levels that directly stimulate the nerves that govern blood vessels, forcing dilatation and swelling and provoking my patient's discomfort and pain.

Effect of Allergic Illness on Smooth Muscle

Blood vessels are not the only body tissue involved in allergic illnesses. Smooth muscle also participates.

THE SAME MECHANISM. Allergy's effect on smooth muscle is the same as on blood vessels. Like the vessels, smooth muscle is richly supplied with nerves, and these nerves "drive" smooth muscle like we drive a car. Also like blood vessels, nerve impulses force smooth muscle to spasm or relax. Unlike the vessels, which cause allergic illness by relaxation (swelling), allergic suffering occurs when smooth muscle spasms or contracts. The smooth muscles we are concerned with encircle the digestive tract and the airways of the lung.

ASTHMA. In looking at asthma, we saw that blood vessel swelling in the lining of the airways constricts the air passages, obstructing the flow of air and causing the whistling or wheezing sound we hear as the air forces itself out of these narrowed air passages. But we shouldn't limit our discussion to swelling of the lining because it is not the only reason the air passages constrict.

Each passage is surrounded by layers of muscle, called smooth muscle, like the water running to a sprinkler is surrounded by the walls of a hose. Unlike the rigid walls of a hose, the muscle around the air passages is alive and in constant motion, contracting and dilating to open or close the numerous branches of the airway, directing the flow of air to different parts of the lung like a traffic officer directs the flow of traffic through a busy intersection.

What if during the rush hour, the traffic officer went on strike, closing half of each road leading into the intersection? Pandemonium would result, with angry, snarling drivers trapped in a gridlock. The stream of traffic would be slowed almost to a halt, and it would take forever for the cars to thread their way through the intersection.

Asthma is like that. Things go smoothly when the airway muscle is functioning normally, contracting and relaxing as it calmly directs the flow of air. When the muscle is in spasm during an asthma attack, the airway narrows, restricting the flow of air through every intersection of the lung.

Food allergy is only one of many causes of asthma attacks, but when the diet is involved, the most likely reason is nerve malfunction signaling the smooth muscle of the airways to go into spasm. Dietary discretion can control this spasm the same way it controls the blood vessel swelling in the lining of the airway.

SMOOTH MUSCLE SPASM ALONG THE DIGESTIVE TRACT. Spasm in the esophagus, one of the first muscles to come in contact with dietary chemicals, causes a distressing **chest pain** similar to the pain that accompanies angioedema as well as to that associated with heart attack. Spasm can also cause transient **difficulties in swallowing**. My patients frequently experience these symptoms.

When such pain occurs in the stomach, it is referred to as **acid stomach** and often leads patients to suspect that they have an ulcer. Those who do have ulcers are especially susceptible to this condition, another example of allergy preying upon an already weakened area. The combination of food allergy and ulcer produces a persistent, knawing pain. Unfortunately, changing the diet will not cure an ulcer, but it can eliminate this aggravating complication.

At the end of the intestine, and surrounded by the same smooth muscle, is the colon, an organ frequently affected by allergy. Here muscle spasms give rise to the **abdominal cramps and diarrhea** that so often make my patients' lives miserable. **Spastic colon** is a frequent diagnosis given to my patients. In most cases, food allergy is not suspected; however, the effects of spastic colon are usually alleviated by changing the diet.

I first encountered this problem years ago in a sensitive and proud woman whose life was terribly affected by diarrhea. Whenever she and her husband went out with friends to dinner and a show, they went an hour early. The reason? She would have an hour-long bout with diarrhea immediately following the meal. Before they could proceed to the theater, her husband and their companions had to wait patiently while she suffered through what must have been a very mortifying situation.

I still remember her sad story, and I regret that I didn't understand food allergy then as well as I do now. At the time, I didn't know how to control her diarrhea.

Allergic Illness—Contact Dermatitis

Our trip through the digestive tract ends at the rectum, where an uncommon but miserable effect of food chemicals manifests itself. A small number of allergy-prone adults complain of an intense **rectal itching** that mystifies doctors. The acidic foods seem unusually adept at causing this uncomfortable and embarrassing condition, although the other chemicals also contribute. **Diaper rash** in babies is more common and is often caused by these same offenders. I suspect that as the stool passes through the anus, the high concentration of diet chemicals it contains irritate and burn the skin. We know this contact reaction occurs at the other end of the body, where our patients suffer a **scalp rash** marked by itching and sores from using shampoos that contain citrus. (I am not sure of the propriety of discussing scalp and rectal rashes in the same paragraph, but they are related.)

Another form of contact dermatitis that should be mentioned is the oh-so-common **hand dermatitis**, sometimes called housewife's hand dermatitis. Anyone who handles acidic foods is susceptible. Contact with these foods reinforces the dermatitis-producing effect of consuming food chemicals (making hands red, dry, cracked, and pathetically itchy).

Allergic Illness—The Central Nervous System

The effect of food allergy on the central nervous system (the brain) is perhaps the most difficult subject to discuss because it is surrounded by uncertainty and controversy. Many doctors and laypeople do not accept the idea that food chemicals can impair brain function or be responsible for the many symptoms our patients suffer. They believe anxiety, depression, and other mood disorders are more likely to be at the root of these symptoms.

I disagree. As we examined our modern diet, we found that certain components are known neurotoxins (aspartic and glutamic acids) and saw how they and their fellow rogue chemicals can generate allergic disease through injury to nerves. Do we suddenly reverse our thinking when it comes to the major nerve center of the body, the brain? I see no reason to do so.

At the same time, I don't want you to think that food chemicals are solely or even primarily responsible for these disorders. Anxiety and psychological instability may be major causes, or they may be contributing factors that potentiate allergy's harm. However, in many cases, food allergy seems to drive these illnesses like a hammer drives a nail, while in other cases, it seems to play more of a supportive role, like the fingers holding the nail. But whatever the relative contribution of each factor, the important thing is to gain relief for my patients, and I find that changing the diet often provides that relief.

A Patient's Story

Perhaps the best way to illustrate the effects of food allergy on mental function is through one of my patient histories. Frequently I see patients who complain of allergic symptoms that are so minor I wonder why they came, but when I ask them how they feel in general, the real reason comes tumbling out. They tell me about being tired, irritable, and depressed all the time—just plain feeling crummy and unable to cope with everyday life. Jackie is one of those patients.

A woman in her forties, Jackie is a middle manager in a nationally known company. She had been feeling tired and listless for so long she was worried about her ineffectiveness at work. "I had my doctor check my thyroid because I was sure I was hypothyroid, but the tests were normal. Then I began to think that I was 'wimping out'—that the tiredness was all in my head."

"That's not at all unusual, Jackie," I assured her. "It isn't necessarily all in your head. Many people find physical factors, such as food allergy, cause these symptoms."

Jackie's symptoms are as frequent in my patients as stuffy nose or headache. What's more, patient's often hide these symptoms as they would hide a disgraceful family secret. Like Jackie, they are afraid to "wimp out" because they don't want to be thought of as a hypochondriac—a whiner and a complainer. They are not any of these things. **Tiredness, irritability,** and often **hyperactivity** (the inability to concentrate) are very real, very common companions of food allergy and usually respond to diet changes.

When Jackie returned to my office after her first three months of treatment to tell me what happened when she changed her diet, we had the following conversation.

"How are you doing, Jackie?"

"Changing my diet helped much more then I thought it would, Doctor Walsh," she reported. "I know you asked me to retry the foods I've eliminated, but I feel so good, I'm afraid to return to them."

"How has the diet made a difference?" I asked.

"I'm surprised at how much better I feel. I'm not as tired, and I've got a lot more ambition at work. Although I'm not a hundred percent better, I have improved so much I no longer think it's all in my head."

Then Jackie told me about another interesting discovery she had made. "I was talking to one of my coworkers the other day. She told me she sees you, too, and has to follow the same diet. Every time she cheats, she ends up feeling tired and irritable and unproductive at work."

Since then, Jackie has found that her ability to concentrate at work is also affected when she strays from the diet, a symptom shared by many of my patients. They have a hard time describing this familiar result of exposure to dietary chemicals, but many agree that an appropriate label would be **"spacy" thinking**.

I know you might think this is going too far—that foods we have eaten all our lives can't possibly affect our mental ability—but don't be too sure. We are learning that the thought and memory processes that take place in the brain are assisted and influenced by neurotransmitters. It does not require a great stretch of imagination to reason that the *neurostimulatory* and *neurotoxic neurotransmitter* chemicals in our modern diet may muddle our thinking and turn it "spacy."

Neurotransmitters are a hot research topic in the study of **depression**. Since allergy and depression are both frequent in the population, it isn't surprising that they often coexist in our patients. Food allergy does not cause depression, but the tiredness, irritability, and ineffective thinking that often accompany it can make depression much harder to overcome. Modifying the diet can help tremendously. Depressed patients who also happen to be allergy-prone deserve the same care as those who are free of this debilitating illness.

Other Allergic Illnesses

Although I have described many of my patient's discomforts and pains, there are still many others I have not included. Every day patients tell me of aches, pains, and discomforts brought on by allergy, many strange and unusual, all a burden. The reason I have not mentioned them is not that they are unimportant, but that there are so many.

Putting Food Allergy in Perspective

What if the president of the United States were to suddenly address the nation in these words:

> "My fellow Americans, our country faces a crisis of unimaginable severity. Not enough scientists and engineers are being trained to design the new machines our modern age demands, or to run the factories that manufacture those machines. Because we lack people who are trained in these skills, we are falling behind competitively in the world marketplace. This must change.

> "Therefore, Congress has passed into law, and I have signed, an emergency measure to reverse this unacceptable situation. From now on, all children will study to be engineers and scientists. The only courses offered in grade school, high school, and college will be math and science. No more English, history, social studies, or business classes will be allowed."

Can you imagine the outrage this misguided proclamation would be greeted with? No doubt a whole new protest movement would form overnight, and with good reason. We all know that not everyone has the talent or the inclination to be an engineer or a scientist, and that our society could not prosper without writers, historians, social scientists, or business experts. It would be a mistake to force everyone into the same profession.

Surprisingly, this scenario has great pertinence to my patients and their food allergies. Just as it is a mistake to think that all children are alike, it is wrong to think that all patients are alike, or to think that all allergic illnesses are identical.

Each patient is a special individual with a distinctive illness that is not like any other patient's illness. For instance, food allergy is an overwhelmingly important cause of headache or wheezing for some patients; for others, food allergy is only a minor contributing factor. Some patients may react badly to one food, while others may be able to tolerate that same food but will have a severe reaction to another food. To keep food allergy in perspective, a doctor must remember these differences in patients, illnesses, and causes. To do otherwise would be a great mistake.

How does a doctor or layman approach the diagnosis and treatment of food allergy and keep it in perspective? I do it by following a number of principles I have learned over many years from the magnificent patients who worked with me to control their discomfort and pain. Each patient's problems and response to treatment helped to slowly open the door to the secrets of allergy. (Perhaps the door will never be fully open, nor the secrets fully revealed.) Let's look at the principles I use to put food allergy in perspective.

NO ILLNESS IS ALLERGY UNTIL IT IS DIAGNOSED AS SUCH BY YOUR PRIMARY PHYSICIAN. Not all illness is due to allergy. You do not need an allergist to do skin tests for your headaches if they are due to a brain lesion, or skin testing for diarrhea if you have bowel disease. Go to your primary doctor for diagnosis. Go to an allergist only after obtaining a proper primary diagnosis.

A NONALLERGIC ILLNESS DOES NOT PRECLUDE ALLERGY. This principle is not a contradiction of the first one. I treat many patients with brain lesions for the allergic component of their headaches, and I help patients with bowel inflammation alleviate the part of their cramps and diarrhea that is caused by allergy. They deserve the same care as any other allergic patient.

NEVER IGNORE ENVIRONMENTAL ALLERGY IN DIAGNOSING FOOD ALLERGY. It is best to assume (and probably true) that all patients react to both foods and to the dust, mold, pollen, and pets in their environment. Patients both breathe and eat; to focus on one to the exclusion of the other means the patient's illness will not be fully evaluated. It is tempting to focus only on food allergy when investigating the allergic reactions of some patients. For example, we often see patients who react to a specific food (i.e., shrimp) in a specific way (i.e., hives). The obvious diagnosis is food allergy, solo and uncomplicated.

Not necessarily. To understand this point, visualize a patient as a bucket you want to fill. If the bucket is already full, any added water will slop over the side. If it's empty, you can add a lot of water before it spills over. The water represents food allergy, and the water spilling over the side is the allergic reaction. Sometimes a patient's food allergy is super strong, and just like adding water to a bucket that is filled to the brim will always cause it to overflow, eating the offending food will always lead to a reaction. All by itself.

At other times, the food allergy is only moderately—or even mildly—strong (like a cup of water poured into the bucket). The patient must be primed or prepared to react before the food can cause trouble, just as the bucket must be almost full before water spills over the side.

This principle explains why food allergy is so frequently intermittent. On a particular day, sugar provokes a migraine; on another day, no headache. Perhaps on the day of the headache, the patient was exposed to a large amount of dust while cleaning out the basement, plus the ragweed pollen count was high. In this example, environmental allergy primed my patient for a headache brought on by sugar, a headache that would not occur on a day with low dust and ragweed exposure.

Dust, mold, and pollen often prime patients to react to foods. That's why categorizing any food allergy as "solo and uncomplicated" is frequently a mistake if environmental allergy is ignored. Foods are usually not the only cause of allergy, even in cases where the evidence points overwhelmingly in that direction.

NEVER IGNORE FOOD ALLERGY IN DIAGNOSING ENVIRON-MENTAL ALLERGY. This principle goes hand in hand with the previous one. Just as it is a mistake to ignore the influence of the environment on food allergy, it is also a mistake to ignore the influence of foods on environmental allergy. Patients suffer if their doctor errs in either direction.

But what about the patient with solo, uncomplicated pollen allergy, the patient who sneezes only during the grass pollen season? Surely foods aren't the cause of this sneezing.

For an answer, let's pretend the allergic patient must carry his allergies around in a bucket. For many, grass (or tree or ragweed) pollen allergy fills the bucket to overflowing. But is the overflow a trickle, or is it a flood? If the patient's bucket is empty of any other allergy, chances are it's a trickle. But if the bucket is partially filled with food allergies, even though the bucket doesn't overflow during the pollen-free months, when the pollen allergy is added, there is likely to be a flood. Similarly, my patients with pollen allergy can be far more uncomfortable if they eat certain foods when the pollen count is high.

Allergy to the food chemicals is so common in our patients that my nurses and I routinely look for them when we investigate problems due to pollen, dust, mold, and pet allergy. The single act of changing the diet during the time my patient is suffering from something in the environment often determines the success or failure of our treatment. It can change a flood of allergy misery into a trickle of discomfort, a miserable pollen season into one that is merely uncomfortable.

EXPLORE BOTH FOOD AND ENVIRONMENTAL ALLERGY IN EVERY PATIENT. This principle reinforces the previous two. A patient is ill served by the doctor who ignores food allergy and concentrates on environmental causes such as pollen, dust, mold, and pets, or vice versa. Breathing and eating are so basic to our existence that factors which affect either area can be equally detrimental to our quality of life. Therefore, it is essential to question the influence of the pollen season on food allergy and of food sensitivity on pollen allergies. Patients deserve these answers.

ATTACK OVERPOWERING FOOD ALLERGY BY ATTACKING ENVIRONMENTAL ALLERGY. Often a patient's food allergies are uncomplicated and easy to diagnose, and avoidance of one or several foods solves the problem neatly. However, sometimes patients are allergic to so many foods and suffer such devastating reactions, I feel almost powerless to help them.

Many examples spring to mind—patients with food allergy so universal they are allergic to practically every food and beverage in our modern diet. Some of the most tragic and pitiable of these patients are those with bulimia and anorexia nervosa. Their horrendous food allergies make these formidable illnesses even more resistant to treatment.

The only effective way to treat these seemingly hopeless cases of food allergy is to eliminate as many other allergens as possible. Using the analogy of the bucket, if the patient's food allergy causes it to overflow, the logical solution is to ensure the bucket is empty of any other allergic factors to make more room for food allergy. In other words, reduce the flood to a trickle.

In this approach to allergy care, the most important strategy is not the treatment of the food allergy itself but the aggressive treatment of any environmental allergy the patient may have—no matter how small. It is amazing how well this works.

ACID FOODS, MSG, ASPARTIC ACID, AND SUGAR ARE THE MOST IMPORTANT FOOD ALLERGIES. This principle downplays the importance of common food allergies such as milk, wheat, peanut butter, and all the other foods that cause allergic symptoms. Since these food allergies are usually spotted by the patient, parents, or primary doctor, the diagnosis is usually apparent, the treatment is avoidance, and an allergist is seldom needed.

Not so with the patients I see. They are part of an immense group of sufferers who react to multiple foods. Diagnosing them is baffling, treating them is complicated, and the skills of an allergist are usually required. For these patients, the potent and damaging food chemicals are commonly the direct or indirect causes of illness, and treatment will fail unless their use of these chemicals is reduced or eliminated. Only then can their other food allergies be controlled.

The prevalence of these food chemicals in our modern diet and their potential for provoking illness make it essential that allergic patients be knowledgeable about them. Not understanding their importance, where they hide in the diet, and how to avoid them condemns many patients to a life of pain and discomfort. This is so unnecessary.

TEMPER YOUR DIET WITH COMMON SENSE. Between those patients who follow our dietary advice with religious fervor, never deviating, and those who take a more balanced approach, avoiding the excesses that bring on symptoms—and cheating at times, I find I have much more success with the latter. The former will eventually give up the diet because the strain of unswerving adherence is too great.

The patient who takes a more common-sense approach can stay on the diet for life, if necessary. When cheating causes the return of unpleasant symptoms, it reinforces the need for avoiding the offending food and makes following the diet easier. This patient is also flexible enough to relax his or her vigilance as the need becomes less. For instance, if environmental allergies are treated aggressively with avoidance and allergy injections, the need for total avoidance decreases commensurately. Flexibility and common sense make the diet easier to follow.

DON'T BE DISCOURAGED. It is normal to feel discouraged when asked to eliminate foods and beverages you enjoy— and even crave. It takes awhile to get used to the idea, but our patients tell us that after about three years, they usually forget they are on a diet.

It is often said that success breeds success, and it seems that when the diet has the desired effect of reducing or eliminating our patients' symptoms, it is no longer a burden for them to follow it. When we question our patients about what they eat, we find they have no trouble avoiding the excessive sugar, MSG, low-calorie sweeteners, and acidic foods that once seemed so essential. It can be the same for you.

Adult and Child Allergy Elimination Diet

The diet described in this chapter is given to our patients when they are evaluated in our office and found allergic to food chemicals. It summarizes many of the points discussed in previous chapters.

The purpose of this diet is to help ease the discomfort brought on by reactions to foods. To do this, you must learn which foods and beverages make you ill so that you can avoid them. Food allergy is a common problem, and most of our patients suffer from it to a greater or lesser degree. By learning how to control your food allergy you can reduce its impact on your life.

For the majority of our patients, food allergy reactions result from sensitivity to certain chemicals in our modern diet. Each chemical is made of substances normally present in our bodies and, when consumed in low quantities, does not cause illness. However, today's diet encourages excessive consumption of certain chemicals. If you learn to avoid the foods and beverages that contain high levels these chemicals, you can avoid much pain and discomfort.

The Food Chemicals

The food chemicals that concern us are (1) citric acid, which is commonly found in our diet, and less frequently encountered acids such as malic acid, tartaric acid, fumaric acid, and succinic acid; (2) refined sugar; (3) monosodium glutamate (MSG); and (4) aspartic acid, found in the artificial sweetener aspartame and sold under the brand names Equal® and NutraSweet®. (The artificial sweetener saccharin, found in many products, must also be avoided).

Note: Citric acid can also be called citrate or citrus, malic acid can be called malate, tartaric acid can be called tartrate, fumaric acid can be called fumarate, and succinic acid can be called succinate.

The Offending Foods and Beverages

The following foods and beverages contain large quantities of the above chemicals.

THE ACID FOODS AND BEVERAGES. Foods and drinks with high citric and related acids have a citrus or fruity taste. Many are natural—not processed (manufactured). For example, berries, cherries, grapes, and the citrus fruits—oranges, lemons, limes, grapefruit—have naturally high levels of citric acid. Others are processed; a manufacturer will add citric or related acids to a beverage or food to give it a pleasant, fruity taste. This addition is always listed in the ingredients, so watch for the presence of citric acid or less commonly malic, tartaric, fumaric or succinic acid. As mentioned, the acids may also be labeled somewhat differently, with the –ic of citric replaced by –ate, as in sodium or potassium citrate.

If the acid is high on the list of ingredients, the amount in the manufactured food is probably large, so you should avoid eating that product. If the acid is listed toward the end, it is probably present in small amounts and should not bother you. In all cases, let your sense of taste guide you; if it tastes fruity, leave it alone.

The following is a partial list of foods and beverages that contain high amounts of citric acid:

1. Candy, jam, jelly, preserves
2. Carbonated and noncarbonated beverages (soda pop, packaged drink mixes, etc.)
3. Desserts (ice cream, flavored gelatin, pies, puddings, etc.).
4. All fruits and berries listed below:

apricots	grapes	pineapple
blackberries	kiwi	plantains
blue berries	kumquats	plums
cherries	lemons	pomegranates
crab apples	limes	prunes
cranberries	loganberries	raisins
currants	mangos	raspberries
dates	mulberries	rhubarb
figs	nectarines	strawberries
gooseberries	oranges	tangerines
grapefruit		

5. Any fruit juices or juice blends
6. Tomatoes, tomato juice, and tomato-based products
7. All potatoes and potato products (potatoes are acidic)

REFINED SUGAR. Refined sugar is used to sweeten many packaged foods and canned and bottled beverages. It will always be listed on the package, although it is often called by different names: corn syrup, honey, brown sugar, molasses, maple syrup. All are refined sugars and can cause symptoms. You need not pursue a diet completely free of all refined sugar; aim for a diet low enough in refined sugar that your symptoms are not stimulated.

The following is a partial list of foods and beverages high in refined sugar:

1. Candy, jam, jelly, preserves
2. Carbonated and noncarbonated beverages containing sugar
3. Desserts (cakes, cookies, ice cream, flavored gelatin, pies, sweet rolls, presweetened cereals, etc.)

MONOSODIUM GLUTAMATE. High quantities of mono-sodium glutamate are naturally present in foods such as mushrooms, kelp (seaweed), and scallops. It is commonly used in prepared meats such as breakfast sausages, bratwurst, hot dogs, luncheon meats, pot pies, frozen pre-pared entrées, and TV dinners. MSG gives these foods an extra hearty taste that is pleasant to the palate but has unpleasant consequences for many allergy sufferers.

Watch for MSG in soups and breaded products, as well as in many snack foods such as crackers, chips, and nuts. It is also used extensively in Chinese cooking, but usually can be avoided by asking the cook to prepare the meal without monosodium glutamate. MSG is released from protein dur-ing the fermentation of foods and beverages; therefore, expect to find it in cheese, soy sauce, and alcoholic bever-ages.

To determine whether processed foods contain MSG, look for it on the label. If you see it listed, do not buy the product. Sometimes MSG is hidden under the catchall phrase "natural flavors"; short of writing to the manufac-turer to ask if the "natural flavors" include MSG, there is no way to be sure whether it is present. Even more frequently, it is disguised by being labeled "hydrolyzed vegetable pro-tein," which contains ten to forty percent MSG. Do not buy such products.

ARTIFICIAL SWEETENERS. Aspartame (NutraSweet® and Equal®) and saccharin are commonly found in carbonated and noncarbonated diet beverages, diet foods, and low-calorie sweeteners for home use. My patients must avoid them.

Using the Diet

STARTING OUT. How you start the diet depends on the frequency of your symptoms. It does not matter whether these symptoms are a stuffy nose, headaches, hives, asthma, abdominal pains, diarrhea, or any of the numerous other symptoms that plague the allergic patient. If your symptoms occur frequently—daily or weekly—you will be able to judge the effect of avoiding these chemicals immediately. Meticulously avoid foods and beverages prohibited by the diet for two weeks and watch for improvement in your symptoms.

If your symptoms occur less frequently—monthly or less often—you may not be able to learn anything from two weeks of elimination, even if you follow the diet meticulously. If you were symptom-free, there would be no way to tell if the diet worked or if you simply didn't experience any symptoms during those two weeks. Therefore, you need not completely abstain from these foods and beverages; instead, we ask you to reduce their use to avoid their unpleasant consequences.

If your symptoms appear only during one season or time of the year, you will need to follow this diet during that season only. Seasonal allergy often arouses underlying food allergy that can make you miserable.

DURING THE DIET. If your symptoms are frequent, avoiding the above foods and beverages for a two-week period allows you to determine their effect on your symptoms. If you find them reduced in frequency or severity— fewer or less severe headaches, wheezing, rash, or other illness—these foods are probably at least partly to blame for your symptoms.

If your symptoms are infrequent, you need not follow a strict elimination diet; however, you should be aware of these foods because they may be major causes of your troubles. Avoid eating or drinking excessive amounts. When illness strikes, recall what you have eaten for the previous twenty-four hours; you should be able to identify the offending foods and beverages. They are usually the foods and beverages listed above.

TESTING THE DIET. A second step is necessary to make sure the particular foods and beverages you suspect are actually the cause of your discomfort. Return them to your diet; if your symptoms flare on reintroduction, you will be more confident that they are the cause. How you do it is up to you. It is perfectly acceptable to first reintroduce the foods and beverages you miss the most, adding them back carefully in small quantities or all of them at once in large quantities. Adding one food at a time is probably not helpful; it is the total quantity of all these foods and beverages combined in your diet that causes pain and discomfort.

LIVING WITH THE DIET. As you become accustomed to this diet, you will find that you can eat and drink many of the prohibited foods and beverages if you limit the quantities to a level you can tolerate. For instance, you may be able to eat one or two cookies in a day, but not ten. You may tolerate a little ketchup, but not a glass of tomato juice. You may tolerate some cheese, but probably not as much as you would like. Eventually, you should be able to determine your level of tolerance for these foods and beverages, making the diet less onerous and you more comfortable.

What You Can Eat

A MENU. The following is menu of foods that are generally acceptable for patients who must avoid certain foods and beverages because of sensitivity. To help plan your menu, we listed some name brands of products we believe are low in chemicals that trouble our patients. We regret this is only a partial list; many good products are not listed.

BREAKFAST

Cereals (use any of the following with milk)

Cheerios	Malt-O-Meal	Rice Krispies
Cream of Rice	Oatmeal	Shredded Wheat
Cream of Wheat	Puffed Rice	Wheat Chex
GRAPE-NUTS Flakes	Puffed Wheat	

BREAKFAST cont.

Eggs
Bacon, ham
Toast with butter or margarine

LUNCH

Grain products (may be used at any meal)

Baking powder biscuits	Muffins (banana, bran, free of citric acid and low in sugar)
Breads (rye, wheat, rice)	
Crackers	
Croissants (plain)	Noodles and macaroni
Flat breads	Rice (white rice, wild rice, rice cakes)
Flour tortillas	

The following are lunch suggestions:

- Sandwich with beef, pork, fish or fowl. Butter or margarine are allowed; may be garnished with lettuce or a pickle.
- Salad with oil and vinegar (not wine vinegar), olive oil, or mayonnaise without lemon juice or citrus added. Lettuce, spinach, onion, carrots, cucumbers, radishes, olives, celery. Accompany with any of the allowed fruits.
- Sausage, hamburgers or hot dogs are allowed if free of added MSG, citrus, or other chemicals.

DINNER

Meat—beef, pork, fish, fowl

Salad—same as lunch salad

Grain products—same as for lunch

Vegetables (any of the following):

artichokes	celery
asparagus	okra
beets	olives (without pimento)
boiled broccoli	parsnips
boiled cabbage	radishes
boiled corn	rutabaga
boiled green beans	squash
carrots	turnips

Fruits—you may have two or more servings of:

apples	peaches
bananas	pears
cantaloupe	watermelon
muskmelon	

Beverages

coffee	unflavored bottled water
milk	water
tea	

Snacks—any crackers or pretzels processed without MSG, sugar, or acids; any nuts without additives other than salt: almonds, Brazil nuts, cashews, filberts, hazelnuts, macadamia nuts, pecans, pistachios, sunflower seeds, walnuts.

ACCEPTABLE FOODS BY FOOD GROUP. The following is a partial list of foods that are acceptable for patients on our diet. The foods are classified according to biologic relationship with examples of each group. *If you have a strong allergy to any of these foods (i.e., nuts, fish), you must avoid it—do not use it in the diet.* If you have a weak allergy to some of the foods we list as acceptable, continue to use these foods unless they cause symptoms. Sometimes, eating them one or two days out of three (rotating foods) will allow you to tolerate them.

ANIMAL GROUPS

Amphibians: frogs

Crustaceans: crab, lobster, shrimp

Eggs

Fish: bass, cod, crappie, flounder, haddock, halibut, salmon, scrod, sunfish, trout, tuna, walleye, whitefish

Fowl: chicken, cornish game hen, duck, goose, turkey

Milk products: butter, milk casein (cheese product)

Mollusks: abalone, clams, oysters, snails

Red meat animals: beef, lamb, mutton, pork, veal (roasts, steaks, chops), bacon, ham

PLANT GROUPS

Beech family: beechnut, chestnut

Birch family: filbert, hazelnut

Cashew family: cashew, pistachio

Ginger family: cardamom, ginger

Goosefoot family: beet, spinach, swiss chard

Gourd family: cantaloupe (muskmelon), casaba, cucumber, honeydew melon, pumpkin, squash, watermelon

Grass family: barley, oats, rice, rye, wheat

Laurel family: avocado, bay leaf, cinnamon

Lecythis: Brazil nut

Lily family: asparagus, chives, garlic, leek, onion

Madder family: cottonseed, okra

Mint family: basil, Japanese artichoke, marjoram, mint, oregano, peppermint, sage, savory, spearmint, thyme

Morning glory family: sweet potato, yam

Mustard family: radish, rutabaga, turnip

Myrtle family: allspice

Olive family: olive

Parsley family: caraway, carrot, celeriac, celery, dill, parsley

Pepper family: black pepper

Plum family: almond

Poppy family: poppyseed

Sunflower family: artichoke, Jerusalem artichoke, lettuce, sunflower

Tea family: tea

Walnut family: black walnut, butternut, English hickory nut, pecan

Additional Information

FRUITS. Most of our patients are able to tolerate two or three servings of the recommended fruits, including apples, bananas, cantaloupe, muskmelon, peaches, pears and watermelon. These fruits are lower in acid; avoid the rest.

CHEESE. Many of our patients tolerate only a limited amount of cheese or none at all. Cheese contains MSG; the more aged the cheese, the more MSG it contains.

LEGUMES. Includes beans, peas, peanuts, and soy beans. Sensitivity to these foods varies; you may or may not be able to tolerate them. Storing fresh peas and beans for twenty-four hours before preparing them, boiling them well, and discarding the boiled water helps reduce symptoms in many of our patients.

POTATOES. Potatoes are a special problem. Most of our patients tolerate only a few meals of potatoes per week; others cannot tolerate any potatoes. Use caution and watch your symptoms when you use them in your diet. Boiling them well may be the best way to serve them. Surprisingly, potatoes are closely related to tomatoes.

CORN AND CORN PRODUCTS. Be careful. Corn allergies are common in our patients; perhaps fifty percent react to corn, especially popcorn or corn on the cob. Use caution and watch for symptoms when eating corn products. Cutting corn free from the cob and boiling it well helps many patients tolerate it.

CABBAGE FAMILY. Many patients react poorly to raw cabbage, broccoli, brussels sprouts, and cauliflower but can eat them when boiled until soft.

REFINED SUGAR. Tolerated in small to moderate quantities by many of our patients. If you are moderately sensitive, you should find that honey on bread, a small slice of cake, several cookies, a doughnut or sweet roll, a little pop, or sugar in your coffee can be tolerated. Keep the total amount of refined sugar or honey consumed in a day to a small or moderate quantity.

VINEGAR. Do not use either wine or apple cider vinegar. Use only vinegar made from grain and as small an amount as possible.

VITAMINS AND FOOD SUPPLEMENTS. Stop all vitamins and food supplements during the two-week trial elimination period. Many supplements contain aspartic and glutamic acid (MSG). Vitamin C needs to be combined with citric acid to prevent deterioration.

ALCOHOL. No alcohol should be consumed on the two-week trial elimination.

Living with the Diet

In the preceding chapters, we examined food allergy and explored the evolution of a diet that excludes the most common causes of this affliction. Because of this diet, patients with untreatable allergic illnesses are now treatable. Their illnesses are no longer mysterious; their suffering need no longer be prolonged.

By following the diet, my patients can be free of pain and discomfort. They can look forward to each day with the expectation that they will feel well.

If you share these food allergies, you can also share this same release from illness. The preceding chapters described which foods and beverages cause headaches, rashes, congestion, bloating, tiredness, and the myriad other symptoms food allergy inflicts on the sensitive person. Now you must use this information to change your diet so that you can reach the precious goal of good health.

The chapters that follow are intended to help you do this. They tell you how to apply the information you have learned in shopping for food,preparing meals to eat at home, and selecting foods from the menu when eating in a restaurant.

A word of caution: I am a specialist only in the allergic illnesses, including food allergy. I am not a specialist in low-cholesterol, diabetic, or other diets. If you have a medical condition that requires you to follow a special diet, you will not be able to eat some of the foods I recommend. To obtain help in adapting our diet to your needs, consult your doctor or a competent dietician.

Reading Labels

My nurses and I usually find that our patients are so tired of feeling ill and so determined to lead normal lives again, they are willing to do anything to restore their good health. Even so, they are dismayed to learn of the many changes they must make in their diet and of the many foods and beverages they must avoid.

They have every right to be dismayed at having to give up so many of the foods and beverages they enjoy. And the magnitude of this lifestyle change must become even more apparent after they leave our office and return home to read the labels on the groceries in their cabinets. The foods and beverages they usually buy are no doubt filled with sugar, MSG, citric acids, and low-calorie sweeteners.

As our patients read these labels, they realize that one of the first things they have to change is their shopping habits. They can no longer grab the old familiar products from the grocery shelves. Now they must be careful to choose foods that do not cause pain and discomfort. They must avoid many old favorites and select foods that are low in content or completely free of MSG, citric acid, refined sugar, and low-calorie sweeteners.

And who can blame them for feeling intimidated by the prospect of learning to shop all over again. As children, we learned to shop by accompanying our parents to the grocery store. Back then it was a fun experience, perched up high in the shopping cart's little bucket seat, every once in awhile throwing something in when Mom wasn't watching. But for adults, shopping is no longer fun but a necessary evil (probably because years and pounds prevent us from sitting in the little bucket seat).

Is it worth the trouble for my patients to change their shopping habits, to stand there reading labels in type so small they can barely make it out? That depends. If foods cause such a splitting headache that it feels as if some fiendish mole is digging a tunnel through their brain—it is. If foods cause such terrible cramping that it feels as if a crowd of protesters is marching through their intestines—it is. If foods cause their body to tire and their brain to function ineptly, as if they spent the entire day slogging through a ditch filled with mud—it is.

To help my patients make the necessary lifestyle changes and avoid such pain and discomfort, this chapter and the ones following it will look at ways to identify troublesome foods while shopping, snacking, eating at home, and eating out. We'll start by stressing the importance of reading labels, and then we'll examine a few of the labels found on prepackaged food products.

The Importance of the Label

Allergic patients must choose their foods carefully, which is not always easy. Today shoppers face a bewildering number of choices as they push their shopping carts down grocery aisles lined by an incredible variety of food selections.

While it is not that difficult to stay away from foods we recognize as harmful, such as tomatoes, cheese, and citrus fruits, it is much harder to avoid these foods in prepared food products. In addition, prepackaged foods usually contain troublesome food additives and chemicals. That's why it's so important for allergic shoppers to become knowledgeable about reading food labels. It will help them determine which foods to buy and which to avoid.

The Food and Drug Administration requires food manufacturers to list the ingredients used in the foods they produce. The ingredients are listed in descending order according to the amount the product contains: the ingredient present in the largest amount is listed first, the ingredient present in the second-largest amount is listed next, and so on, until all of the ingredients are listed according to the quantity present in the food.

The list of ingredients is a valuable guide for food-sensitive people. Reading the label is the best way to avoid those foods that cause unacceptable symptoms.

As I mentioned earlier, some of my patients find they tolerate certain chemicals such as sugar and the citrus or fruit acids if they are present in small quantities. In this case, the foods will not have a strong sweet or fruity taste and the sugar or acid will be listed near the end of the list of ingredients. Therefore, if an ingredient such as sugar or citric acid is listed far down the list of ingredients, the food may be acceptable while following our diet.

Unfortunately for many of my patients, they cannot tolerate even small quantities of MSG and low-calorie sweeteners. For them, foods containing MSG and low-calorie sweeteners must be avoided entirely, along with foods with pronounced sweet or fruity flavors.

Some Example Labels

To illustrate the various terms used by food processors, I have reproduced the lists of ingredients for several types of prepackaged foods. When the list of ingredients contains chemicals that are poorly tolerated by my patients, they are highlighted to call your attention to them. Patients with food allergy should avoid eating foods with these ingredients. If no ingredients are highlighted, the foods are acceptable.

SPAGHETTI NOODLES

INGREDIENTS: SEMOLINA, NIACINAMIDE, FERROUS SULFATE (IRON), THIAMINE MONONITRATE AND RIBOFLAVIN.

Note: Contains no problem ingredients.

COMPLETE BUTTERMILK PANCAKE MIX

INGREDIENTS: BLEACHED ENRICHED FLOUR [(BLEACHED FLOUR, MALTED BARLEY FLOUR, NIACIN, IRON, THIAMINE, MONONITRATE (VITAMIN B1), RIBOFLAVIN (VITAMIN B2)], YELLOW CORN FLOUR, **SUGAR**, **DEXTROSE**, BAKING POWDER (BAKING SODA, MONOCALCIUM PHOSPHATE, SODIUM ALUMINUM PHOSPHATE), BUTTERMILK, SALT, EGG WHITES, MONO AND DIGLYCERIDES, NONFAT MILK, LECITHIN, EGGS, HYDROGENATED SOYBEAN OIL, **CORN SYRUP SOLIDS**.

The various forms of sugar have been highlighted in the above ingredient list. Refined sugar can be a problem for many people if it is consumed in too large a quantity. Unfortunately, the Food and Drug Administration does not require food processors to include on the label what percentage of the total product content is accounted for by a particular ingredient. Instead, ingredients are listed in descending order of content, with the ingredient accounting for the highest percentage of the total product listed first.

In the pancake mix above, sugar is the third ingredient, listed, dextrose is the fourth, and another form of sugar— corn syrup solids—ends the list. Although the label does not tell us what percentage of the total content these sugars represent, this mix probably contains too much sugar for patients on our diet. If the item tastes sweet, you should not eat it; no matter where it is listed in the ingredient list, the sugar content is probably too high.

SKILLET HAMBURGER MIX

INGREDIENTS: ENRICHED MACARONI, VEGETABLE SHORT-ENING (CONTAINS ONE OR BOTH OF THE FOLLOWING PARTIALLY HYDROGENATED OILS: SOYBEAN, COTTONSEED), **CHEDDAR CHEESE**, (MILK, SALT, CHEESE CULTURES, ENZYMES, COLOR ADDED), CORN STARCH, **TOMATO** (WITH COLOR PROTECTED BY SODIUM BISULFITE), BUTTERMILK, SALT, **SUGAR**, **HYDROLYZED VEGETABLE PROTEIN**, ONION, **CORN SYRUP**, DISODIUM PHOSPHATE (FOR SMOOTH SAUCE), GARLIC, **NATURAL FLAVORS**, **SODIUM CASEINATE** (A MILK PROTEIN), **CITRIC ACID**, (FOR FLAVOR), DIPOTASSIUM PHOSPHATE (FOR SMOOTH SAUCE), YELLOW 5 AND YELLOW 6.

Don't use this mix. Not only does it contain cheese, tomato, hydrolyzed vegetable protein, corn syrup, natural flavors, and citric acid, it also contains sodium caseinate. Casein is made by precipitating it from skim milk by the addition of an acid, a process similar to the one used in cheesemaking. In the diet, it can cause the same problems as cheese. This product contains too many ingredients that are troublsome.

CHICKEN COATING MIX

INGREDIENTS: BLEACHED BROMATED WHEAT FLOUR, **DEXTRIN** (FROM CORN), PARTIALLY HYDROGENATED SOYBEAN AND COTTONSEED OILS, SALT, PAPRIKA, MALTED BARLEY, SPICES (MUSTARD FLOUR, CELERY SEED, CHILI PEPPER, BLACK PEPPER, THYME, BASIL, RED PEPPER, CLOVES, OREGANO, ROSEMARY), **SUGAR**, YEAST, BEET POWDER (FOR COLOR), GARLIC POWDER, ONION POWDER, **NATURAL HICKORY SMOKE FLAVOR**, TBHQ AND CALCIUM PROPIO-NATE (TO PRESERVE FRESHNESS).

This coating mix does not contain MSG or hydrolyzed vegetable protein (except perhaps in the natural hickory smoke flavor), but it does contain sugars. If you use it, you may experience discomfort, especially if other poorly toler-ated foods are consumed in the same time period.

CANNED MEAT

INGREDIENTS: CHOPPED PORK SHOULDER MEAT WITH HAM MEAT ADDED AND SALT, WATER, SUGAR, SODIUM NITRATE.

CHICKEN FLAVOR RICE MIX

INGREDIENTS: ENRICHED EGG WHITE MACARONI PRODUCT, **NATURAL FLAVORS**, SALT, PARTIALLY HYDROGENATED VEGETABLE OIL (SOYBEAN AND OR COTTONSEED), FOOD STARCH, **MODIFIED CORN SYRUP**, **SUGAR**, CHICKEN, **MONOSODIUM GLUTAMATE**, ONIONS, MODIFIED VEGETABLE GUM, **SODIUM CASEINATE**, GARLIC, YEAST, CHICKEN BROTH, SOY FLOUR, PARSLEY, SPICE, DISODIUM INOSINATE, DISODIUM GUANYLATE.

Because this mix contains MSG (monosodium glutamate), as well as sodium caseinate and sugars, avoid using it. The combination of these chemicals is likely to cause problems. Note that the term "natural flavors" is also listed. There is no way of knowing whether this term includes MSG.

GELATIN DESSERT

INGREDIENTS: **SUGAR**, GELATIN, ADIPIC ACID (FOR TARTNESS), DISODIUM PHOSPHATE (CONTROLS ACIDITY), **FUMARIC ACID** (FOR TARTNESS), ARTIFICIAL COLOR, ARTIFICIAL FLAVOR.

Note: This product is probably too sweet.

INSTANT PUDDING

INGREDIENTS: **SUGAR, DEXTROSE (CORN SUGAR)**, CORN STARCH MODIFIED, SODIUM PHOSPHATES (FOR PROPER SET), SALT, HYDROGENATED SOYBEAN OIL WITH BHA (PRESERVATIVE), DI AND MONOGLYCERIDES (PREVENT FOAMING), NONFAT MILK, ARTIFICIAL COLOR (INCLUDING YELLOW 5 AND YELLOW 6), ARTIFICIAL AND **NATURAL FLAVOR**.

Note: Contains too much sugar.

TUNA IN SPRING WATER

INGREDIENTS: CHUNK LIGHT TUNA IN SPRING WATER, VEGETABLE BROTH, SALT, **HYDROLYZED PROTEIN**.

Note: Don't use this product.

FRUIT JUICE

INGREDIENTS: **GRAPE, APPLE AND PASSION FRUIT JUICES**, FROM CONCENTRATES, **NATURAL FLAVOR**, VITAMIN C.

Note: This product is probably too acidic; don't use it.

PEAR HALVES IN HEAVY SYRUP

INGREDIENTS: PEARS, WATER, **CORN SYRUP** AND .

Note: May be used if syrup is rinsed off thoroughly.

Label reading is a skill developed over time. If you eat or drink something that causes you to experience symptoms, check the label; the product may contain an item not acceptable on the elimination diet. As you learn to recognize the problematic food additives and chemicals by name, it will be easier to avoid buying products that contain them.

Is This Too Much To Expect?

Will our patients be able to make this change in shopping habits? Yes, I believe they can. Will the sacrifices they make—eliminating favorite foods and beverages—be more than they can stand? Not when they begin to feel better. They will choose to follow the diet because they are not quitters. They have already proven this by refusing to accept their illness as something they cannot conquer, something they cannot understand, or something they cannot treat.

By coming to our office for treatment, they have demonstrated their commitment to doing whatever is necessary to understand and overcome their illness. Like so many patients before them, they are willing to tolerate a wrench-ing diet change to be free of pain and discomfort, bloating and achiness, and chronic tiredness, to live normally. They are winners, and although I am always sympathetic to their plight, I am also proud of their strength and determination.

Shopping for Groceries

To avoid eating foods that cause illness, our patients' need to practice wise food selection. The best way to prevent eating harmful foods is not to have such foods on hand. This means carefully reading the labels on foods at the grocery store.

Unfortunately, checking the ingredients of every item makes grocery shopping more complicated. When we recommend this to our patients, we're often asked, "Exactly how should I select foods at the store?" I decided that the best way to answer this question was to put myself in their place, so I made I trip to the grocery store.

Since I share my patients' food sensitivity and must continually examine what I buy, it was easy for me to imagine the problems my patients experience as they shop. Perhaps my observations from that excursion will serve as a guide for them as they learn to cope with a new way of shopping.

Cereals

As I pushed my cart through the door of the grocery store, I entered the cereal section, with its confusing array of brightly colored boxes. *What better place to start shopping,* I thought.

Ignoring the sugar-coated cereals for obvious reasons, I examined the rest. One after another, I read the lists of ingredients. On many of the uncoated cereals, sugar was listed as the second or third ingredient—and some listed two or even three types of refined sugar under such names as brown sugar, corn syrup, honey, and so on. Although the cheerful box designs are pleasing, for my sugar-sensitive patients the contents are not. They would tolerate these cereals poorly.

It was only later, in a less prominent part of the store, that I found the low-sugar cereals my patients can tolerate—the Puffed Rice, Puffed Wheat, Rice Krispies, and Shredded Wheat. Also in this section were the boxes of Cream of Wheat and plain oatmeal that I eat (flavored oatmeal may contain sugar and citrus). I suspect that these low-sugar cereals are not displayed on the heavily traveled aisles because they are far less popular and less frequently purchased than the sugared cereals.

This seems like a good place to reinforce an important point for my patients to remember. If they select cereals with a delicious, sweet taste, they will undoubtedly have a high sugar content. If they select cereals with a refreshing fruity taste, they will contain high amounts of citric, malic, and fumaric acids.

Flavored cereals are nutritious foods and perfectly fine to eat unless the fruit flavorings cause noses to stuff up or skin to itch and break out in large, red, blotchy hives. A breakfast of high-sugar cereal is fine unless it causes throats to hurt, voices to turn raspy, or breathing to become labored. Although these cereals have a delightful taste, the aggravating symptoms they cause for the food-sensitive person will soon outweigh any enjoyment. Should my patients eat them? For people who suffer these onerous allergic symptoms, the answer is no.

The Fruit Section

Next I entered the fruit section of the store. In the citrus display, the oranges and grapefruit seemed to radiate an irresistible attractiveness, tempting me to buy and enjoy them. However, if I did, the acid factory in my stomach would go on overtime, sending its hydrochloric acid product burning painfully down my intestines and up my esophagus. Regretfully, I passed by these handsome fruits.

The muskmelons and watermelons looked equally inviting and delicious. The bananas almost glowed with ripeness, and the bright red apples looked as healthy as the blush on the cheek of a child playing in the winter snow. The pears were full and ripe, the peaches swollen with juice. Thankfully, these lower acid fruits are acceptable on our diet.

I am not sure why apples and pears are so well tolerated by my patients. Both contain lots of malic acid, so I suspect that malic acid is better tolerated then the other fruit-derived citric acids.

The Vegetable Section

Patients following our diet should find selecting vegetables easier than selecting fruits, with the exception of the nightshade family of vegetables. The tomatoes, potatoes, eggplant, and red and green peppers that make up this family carry too high a content of MSG and citric acid, so these vegetables must be avoided. It is especially hard to tell my patients they must give up potatoes because so many of us are accustomed to including them with our meals almost daily. Fortunately, rice and pasta make good substitutes for this problematic food.

As I proceeded through the vegetable section, I spotted many acceptable salad ingredients. All varieties of lettuce and spinach are tolerated, as well as carrots, celery, radishes, and onions. Mixed with sunflower seeds and ripe olives, these vegetables make a tasty salad that is whole-some and nutritious. Unfortunately, I am still unsure what salad dressing to advise (that's why I eat my salad without dressing). Grain-based or white vinegar and oil dressing is probably acceptable for those who cannot eat salad without dressing. Salad dressings loaded with tomato, citrus, fruit juice, and sugar are not acceptable.

While I'm on the subject of salads, a word of warning: Be cautious of croutons. Although they add a gratifying crunchiness to a salad, many brands contain MSG or dried cheese (cheese contains MSG) and can trouble my MSG-sensitive patients.

As I continued through the vegetable section, I came to the cabbage family display—solid, leafy green heads of cabbage nestled together, darker green Brussels sprouts that so resemble their larger relatives, cauliflower looking like snow-white flowers snipped from their stems, and broccoli looking like bouquets of flowers picked before they opened. Each of these vegetables is a valuable part of a meal. Many of my patients can eat vegetables of the cabbage family either raw or cooked, but some have trouble and must either avoid them or boil them well before eating.

Later, in the freezer section, I spotted many vegetable selections that are acceptable for my food-sensitive patients—fresh frozen peas, beans, corn, carrots, broccoli, cauliflower, and onions in various combinations. Most of my patients tolerate these frozen vegetables; those with minor sensitivity can serve them steamed, but those who are more sensitive will need to boil them well. Avoid mix-tures containing green and red peppers and mushrooms.

I passed by the selections of frozen vegetables in sauce without stopping. MSG, cheese, or refined sugar is often used to make these pleasing sauces, and although many people can tolerate these flavoring agents, they are not well tolerated by my patients.

Regretfully, I also passed by a food I love to eat—corn on the cob. I don't know what divine purpose is served by instilling in us an overpowering craving for the foods that cause pain. I do know that I and many of my patients experience bloating and abdominal discomfort from eating this delicious late-summer treat, and we had best stick to corn cut from the cob and boiled.

Many other vegetables may be acceptable for patients on our diet—vegetables I have not learned to eat and thus do not fully appreciate. I hope to include them in the future.

The Meat Section

UNPROCESSED MEAT (PLAIN MEAT WITHOUT ADDED FLAVORINGS). Busy days at the grocery store have always reminded me of the bumper-car ride at an amusement park, and this day was no exception, but I finally made it to the meat section. For food allergy sufferers, beef, pork, lamb, chicken, turkey, and fish are a godsend because few patients react badly to them. Unfortunately, a few unlucky souls show a positive skin test to these meats and tolerate them poorly, especially fish, which cause hives in some patients. However, in general, they are acceptable for most food-sensitive people.

Which meats are okay to purchase? Any of the unprocessed cuts of beef, such as roasts or steaks (my vote goes to the delicious T-bone). Thinly sliced roast beef for sandwiches is probably acceptable, as long as the preparation did not include a marinade that contains MSG, such as wine or soy sauce. Steak sauce is a no-no, as it is likely to contain poorly tolerated ingredients.

Unprocessed pork chops, roasts, and bacon are acceptable, as well as lamb for those who enjoy its flavor. A favorite of mine is leg of lamb, and on this day it seemed particularly hard to resist.

The fish looked superb. I enjoy grilling fish plain or with a little olive oil, salt, and pepper in an open boat shaped from aluminum foil. Salmon grilled this way would be fit for a king (well, maybe not my salmon, but I'll get the hang of it someday).

For my food-sensitive patients, chicken is a great food. I often grill a large number of chicken legs and breasts after removing the skin and then freeze them so they can be reheated in a microwave for quick lunches and dinners. Seasoned with a little salt and pepper, they make a delicious meal free of troublesome flavorings.

Turkey is also an excellent food for my patients, but they must be careful when purchasing whole turkeys. Many have been injected with an MSG-containing flavoring, often hydrolyzed vegetable protein. MSG-sensitive persons must avoid them.

I feel especially sorry for my patients who are vegetarians. Please understand, I think a carefully planned vegetarian diet is a healthy one, but having to avoid meats certainly limits food choices for the vegetarian. To further restrict the vegetarian's already limited diet by eliminating high-acid fruits and vegetables is a hardship, even though the purpose—to prevent pain and discomfort—may be worthy.

PROCESSED MEATS (MEATS TO WHICH FLAVORING HAS BEEN ADDED). With some dread, I entered the section of the grocery store most likely to frustrate my patients. Sandwich meats, breakfast sausages, processed lunch and dinner meats, breaded meat selections, and processed meat in sauces stared back at me in bewildering varieties. These are such a convenience for the busy person—just heat and serve for a meal or slap into a sandwich to eat at work or school. What could be easier?

It's not easy to find processed meats that won't cause headaches or diarrhea in food-sensitive people. It can be a real time-waster—reading label after label searching for those that are free of MSG, excess sugar, and the citric acids—because not many are available.

In processed meats, the most important food chemical to avoid is MSG in all its forms. As I hunted through the selections, I found label after label listing MSG, autolyzed yeast, and hydrolyzed vegetable protein (one label called it hydrolyzed plant protein, which seemed a novel way to describe what was probably MSG).

Many labels list "natural flavorings," and because natural flavorings usually contain MSG, and because MSG is likely to be used in meat preparations because of its ability to enhance the flavor, I consider all selections in the processed meat section to contain MSG if they contain natural flavorings. I eliminate any thought of buying them.

Although small amounts of sugar and citrus can be tolerated by most of my patients, MSG—even in small quantities—is frequently not well tolerated. Having to avoid MSG makes shopping in the processed meat section a real pain for them.

I have been able to simplify shopping for processed meats by finding a few products that are free of MSG and excess sugar and buying only those products. Fortunately, there is a brand of sandwich meats that is acceptable— Louis Rich. I find the turkey preparations delicious, especially the smoked turkey ham and turkey nuggets. On this trip, I noticed another acceptable brand, Mr. Turkey, which advertises on the label that it is free of MSG. The labels on both Mr. Turkey and Louis Rich products do not list any suspicious ingredients, including natural flavorings. Both contain sugar, but I think the amount is small and should be acceptable.

I enjoy the flavor of bratwurst, but I couldn't find any acceptable varieties on this trip. This was not a major inconvenience, because I know of a grocery store that makes its own bratwurst, and the butcher insists it is free of MSG and

MSG-containing flavorings. Since I have eaten it without experiencing any bloating or abdominal pain, I believe him.

After checking the labels on two zillion (a little exaggerated) breakfast sausages, I found two brands that were clearly acceptable. Jones Dairy Farm Little Pork Sausages and Woodend Pork Sausage and Pork Sausage Links. Since breakfast sausages make breakfast a more enjoyabale meal, finding these two brands was a real triumph. Both were deemed excellent in the "Walsh Eat 'Em for Breakfast Taste Test."

The Dairy Section

Choices are relatively simple in the dairy section. Butter and fresh milk are acceptable. Sweet-tasting products, including ice cream, are not—they may contain one of the citric acids or refined sugar. Because it is a fermented product, and because fermentation releases MSG, cheese must be approached with caution. The longer a cheese is aged, the more MSG is released, so some of the aged cheeses have large amounts of MSG.

Between fresh milk and aged cheese there is room for compromise. Less sensitive patients (milder and less frequent symptoms) may tolerate minimally aged cheese products such as American processed cheese or cottage cheese if they do not eat too much (always read the list of ingredients). Since the amount of MSG formed naturally during cheese manufacturing is not listed, eating these cheeses is always chancy. Some brands of plain, unflavored yogurt may be fermented less then others and may be acceptable in moderate amounts for those who consider yogurt important. When my patients ask, I advise them to buy several brands and experiment.

Soups

I enjoy soup but have had difficulty finding one without MSG. They are scarce. During my shopping trip, I noticed that the label on one brand of soup read "No MSG." *Great,* I said to myself. *Finally, a soup I can eat.* No such luck! The label listed several varieties of aged cheese as well as that warning sign, "natural flavoring." Although the manufacturer did not add pure MSG to the soup, it was there in the cheese and maybe in the natural flavoring.

I wonder whether food manufacturers are even aware that aged cheese is one of the richest sources of MSG found in foods. What other reason could there be for adding aged cheese to soup and then proudly claiming it is free of MSG?

This experience prompts me to repeat the three most important shopping instructions for the food-sensitive person: (1) Read the label, (2) read the label, and (3) read the label.

The Health Food Store

Much later, I made a trip to a health food store to see if I could find soups without MSG. I found only one, Hain All Natural Chicken Noodle Soup. The label lists natural flavoring, but a parenthetical following the listing indicates that the natural flavoring is an extract of celery, which hopefully has little or no MSG.

While there, I also found a can of Swanson Premium White and Dark Chunk Turkey in Water. The label lists only turkey, water, and salt. A nice sized can for a turkey salad.

Reflections on Shopping

Choosing foods without MSG, low-calorie sweeteners, excess citrus acids, and excess refined sugar is an effort, but it can be done. I do it and my patients do it. The important thing is not to lose sight of the benefits—food-sensitive patients feel much better if they choose foods they can eat without pain and discomfort.

Remember, always read the label. Food manufacturers can—and do—change ingredients. Sitting in my freezer are two pork sausage preparations that used to be free of MSG.

They now contain it, but I didn't read the labels of these *safe* foods when I bought them. I won't eat them. I should have read the labels.

As I shopped, I was troubled by the many foods that contain small amounts of refined sugar, even some of the foods I have recommended. Remember that famous saying about government spending: "A billion dollars here and a billion dollars there, and soon you are talking about real money." Food allergy is like that. A little sugar here and a little sugar there, and soon my patients are talking about headaches, hives, stuffy noses, and all kinds of other allergy miseries. Watch the sugar. Even the small amounts. If you can, choose foods without any refined sugar.

I did not cover all the food choices my patients face when they shop—many are discussed elsewhere, including the chapter on snacking. Nor have I covered all the acceptable food selections—just those I examined on my trip through the grocery store. But I hope I have provided some helpful ideas for shopping wisely.

My patients are intelligent and determined people who insist on taking control of their health and will do what is necessary to relieve the illnesses that those with less strength and determination—and more self-sympathy— will simply choose to endure. The sacrifices they make are made because they know that the sun shines brighter and the day's triumphs are sweeter when they rid themselves of food-caused suffering.

My patients should understand that they have the power to change the way food is prepared—far more power than anything I may say or write. By buying brands such as Louis Rich, Mr. Turkey, Jones Dairy Farm, and Woodend and leaving products with MSG and natural flavoring on the shelf, they will be sending a clear message to food manufacturers. The law of supply and demand will force these manufacturers to supply more products that are acceptable for people with food sensitivities.

Finally, the fact that I am not a particularly skilled shopper—if I can shop for food, anybody can—became very apparent when I returned from the store and emptied my pockets. I found the coupon I had so cleverly taken to the store to redeem on a purchase. And not so cleverly forgot to hand to the cashier.

Eating at Home

Although my nurses and I know our patients have a good chance of controlling their illnesses by changing their diet, and that they will feel much better if they follow this advice, we also know that they will be disheartened at first. Who can blame them for saying, as so many have, "You're asking me to eliminate all the foods I like to eat." The decision to change your diet so drastically is a difficult one, but the rewards are great: and end to pain and discomfort and the start of brighter, sunnier days filled with the joy and satisfaction of feeling well.

The previous chapter presented some thoughts on shopping for foods that do not contain the dietary chemicals my patients must limit or avoid entirely. In this chapter, I want to share some ideas on how to prepare everyday meals using these foods.

How I Follow the Diet at Home

Being forced to follow the same advice my patients must follow gives me a unique perspective on how to prepare meals while following our diet. I know acceptable meals can be prepared because I prepare them. Each day my food and beverage choices are guided by the diet.

I hope my experiences can be of help to food allergy sufferers as they plan their diet. Please understand that as I describe my diet, I am not including all the foods and beverages that can be used, just those I usually eat and drink.

Breakfast

If there was ever a creature of habit, it is I. For some unknown reason, my stomach wakes me at about five o'clock every morning, telling me to rise and shine—it's hungry! Having a stomach like mine must be like having a dog that scratches on the door early every morning, begging to start the day with a walk and a meal. At least my stomach doesn't bark.

My breakfast certainly shows this same love of habit—I eat the same thing almost every day. Into a small pan goes a cup of oatmeal, a pinch of salt, and a sliced banana—stirred until the oatmeal thickens. A banana may not seem sweet to someone whose diet includes lots of refined sugar, but for those of us who must avoid refined sugar, the taste of a banana mixed with hot oatmeal is like the finest sweet treat (at least to me it is). With a serving of skim milk, I have a breakfast I enjoy.

Unfortunately, not all my patients can eat the same meal every day. We treat many patients with "global" food allergy; they are allergic to every food they eat. Fortunately for these unlucky people, if they change their diet frequently (rotate their foods), they can eat without discomfort. It would be a mistake for them to eat oatmeal every day,as I do, but they can rotate oatmeal with Cream of Wheat, Puffed Rice, Shredded Wheat, or other fine cereals low in sugar and without low-calorie sweeteners or citrus.

I confess that I do not eat oatmeal every day. Once or twice a week, usually on the weekend, I enjoy a delightful breakfast of bacon or sausages with sunny-side-up eggs and pancakes or toast with apple butter. I thoroughly enjoy this meal.

However, if you eat these foods for breakfast, be careful of several important items. Make sure the sausage is free of MSG, hydrolyzed vegetable protein, autolyzed yeast extract, or natural flavorings. Do not use syrup on the pancakes—a little salt or butter or an egg on top of the pancakes will have to serve as your syrup. Do not overdo the apple butter (although I think this spread is better tolerated than the high-sugar or high-citrus jellies and jams). Also, forget the fruit juice; in it is concentrated the fruit's acid.

Lunch

Lunch is not a particularly difficult meal to prepare while following our diet. In my case, ensuring an acceptable meal is made simpler by my habit of taking a brown-bag lunch to the office each day. Eating lunch at my desk gives me time to study and to complete the many tasks necessary to the functioning of an allergy practice while feeding the carpet stray crumbs that fall as I eat. I often wonder if my carpet appreciates the meal it shares with me.

I usually eat the same lunch—whole-grain bread plus lettuce and meat, usually turkey breast or other prepared meats made from turkey—which is fine with me. There is no reason not to use beef or pork-based sliced meat; many are now prepared without MSG-containing flavorings. To find these sandwich meats, spend an hour reading the labels on the sandwich meats at your local grocery—there are selections you can use. This is a great improvement over the few selections available ten years ago, when I started to realize the importance of food allergy and discovered that the hunt for acceptable sandwich meats constituted a tedious task.

An egg salad or tuna salad sandwich also tastes excellent. Be very careful that the tuna salad does not contain MSG or MSG-containing flavoring, often hidden under the term "natural flavorings." Many brands of tuna contain MSG—check the label before buying it (or any food product, for that matter). Remember, if you are sensitive to MSG, any time you avoid buying MSG-containing food, you avoid eating it and spare yourself unpleasant symptoms. You also encourage the food manufacturer to prepare more food products that do not contain it. They will produce products that sell.

Top off the sandwich with a pear or apple to make the meal complete. These fruits travel well in a lunch bag and seem well tolerated on the diet.

On the weekends I fix my own lunch. If I'm in a hurry, I find nothing beats a bagel, warm and smelling fragrantly of fresh-baked bread after a trip to the microwave. It takes just a few more minutes to prepare a frozen chicken leg in the microwave. I keep a supply of chicken legs on hand, prepared by cooking a large number on the grill and basting them on one side with a very light coating of honey (even I cheat on the sugar avoidance at times). Alternatively, they can be prepared in the oven, dusted with a coating of crushed corn flakes.

In either preparation, I always remove the skin before placing the legs in the oven or on the grill. After they cool, each leg is wrapped in aluminum foil, frozen, and saved for a future meal when a quick trip to the microwave provides a nourishing entrée acceptable on our diet.

Another lunch I enjoy is sausage—one of the various types that are free of MSG in any of its forms. As with the chicken, the sausages are precooked, frozen, and heated before finding their way into my sandwich.

Or, if I have the time and ambition, I will make a salad of lettuce, ripe olives, sliced onions, sunflower seeds, and perhaps sliced beef or turkey. I find this salad pleasing to the taste without salad dressing—skipping the salad dressing frees me from trying to find a salad dressing that does not contain sugar, MSG, tomatoes, or vinegar. (Vinegar is a product of fermentation and probably contains a small amount of fermentation-derived MSG. If you must use a vinegar-based dressing, use grain-derived or white vinegar to avoid those made from wine or cider.)

An egg salad or tuna salad prepared with mayonnaise that doesn't contain citrus fruit juice can make a delightful lunch; add onions, celery, and any other ingredients that appeal to your palate. Remember to watch out for MSG in the tuna.

Dinner

The evening meal is a special meal—a time to relax after the hurry and bustle of the day, a time to become reacquainted with the family and share experiences, a time to prepare for the events of the evening, whether these include a social engagement, a task that could not be completed during the day, or a quiet time with a good book.

My patients can enjoy this meal while avoiding the foods and beverages that bring distress. Preparing the meal at home allows them to control its content, something that cannot be done when eating at a restaurant or a friend's home. I suspect this is what encourages my patients to eat at home once they understand which foods and beverages they must avoid. Besides, there is great pride and satisfaction in preparing a delicious home-cooked meal.

One of my favorite dinners features fresh fish of any type, although my palate finds salmon the best tasting. I do not know whether the salmon appreciate this endorsement. Nesting the salmon on a bed of rice, especially wild rice, makes a delectable meal that I enjoy thoroughly. The rice can be prepared by precooking a large amount ahead of time, storing it in the refrigerator, then removing and heating a meal-sized portion for dinner. Packaged rice can also be used, but watch out for MSG flavoring in these products. Using home-prepared rice ensures that it is free of anything that causes discomfort.

If I'm in the mood for beef, a hamburger with lettuce, onions, and sliced pickles satisfies this craving. A nice salad, prepared as described previously, complements the meal. Instead of hamburger, a bratwurst or other sausage without MSG might tempt me. Or, if I want a more substantial piece of beef, I might choose a steak (my favorite is T-bone) broiled in the oven or barbecued on the grill, accompanied by asparagus (in season) or peas or beans, boiled well. Any of these meats is also great with corn sliced from the cob and boiled well. Although corn boiled while still on the cob is a superlative dish, it is also one I regret eating surprisingly soon.

In the mood for pork chops? Shake a few chops in a paper bag containing a mixture of flour and pepper and fry them in a small amount of vegetable oil. The taste is outstanding.

Notice I have not included potatoes in my meals. For me, as for many of my patients, potatoes are too easily eaten in excess. The allergic patient is never sure how much potato can be tolerated without experiencing the same symptoms caused by tomatoes. For many, one or two servings of potatoes per week is no problem, but they find that excess amounts cause discomfort. If a patient is unsure of how much is too much, it is often best not to eat potatoes at all. For those more adventurous than I, enjoy your potatoes but eat them prudently.

Dessert

A sweet treat is a nice reward after a busy and productive day, a satisfying way to end the evening meal. Visions of cherry or lemon meringue pie or any of the exquisite-tasting ice creams, especially those with chocolate, must dance through the dreams of the unfortunate victim of food allergy. I know they dance through the dreams of this victim.

Although I can't enjoy these fine desserts—my body complains loudly for days if I eat them—I have many fond childhood memories of finishing the evening meal with a delicious bowl of ice cream. Since that time I have learned that I must avoid refined sugar. Many of my patients also share this experience. For them, carbonated beverages with low-calorie sweeteners cannot be replaced with beverages containing refined sugar, nor can a dessert of delectable cheesecake be substituted for a slice of sugar-laden pie or cake.

To summarize the role of desserts in our diet—they belong in my patient's dreams and not in their stomachs. Unless someone comes up with a dessert that doesn't contain refined sugar, MSG, low-calorie sweeteners, or citrus-type acids, food-sensitive people must be content with an apple, a pear, a banana, a peach, or a slice of melon. Although these fruits do not have the aroma and flavor of a piping-hot slice of pie or the smooth creaminess of a dish of ice cream, they are a healthy and safe alternative.

A Reflection

I regret that to follow our diet, our patients must eliminate or reduce their consumption of many delicious foods and beverages. But I know that for those with headaches, abdominal cramps, eczema, and many other illnesses, the inconvenience and distress of being on the diet is better than suffering through their painful food reactions. Most of our patients agree and are happy with the results.

Snacks

Our human nature seems to rebel against a rigid schedule of three meals a day. Although we struggle to adapt our digestive system to regular meals, we are not always successful. Like a baby awakening from a nap with an insistent cry of hunger, our stomachs often demand food well before the next meal is due, and we react to this demand by hunting for a snack.

Food manufacturers have responded to this between-meal demand for food by producing a large assortment of products to be eaten for snacks. Individual selections are numerous, and many are irresistibly delicious.

What foods and beverages might be okay for a snack? Imagine yourself rummaging through the kitchen shelves and the refrigerator in search of a between-meal treat. You say to yourself, "My, that ice cream in the freezer looks good. Or those potato chips with that tasty cheese dip—how perfect for a snack. Or shall I choose the flavored corn chips, or those chocolate chip cookies? Maybe I should stick to my diet, peel that juicy orange, and limit the calories and pounds." Of course, a high-citrus carbonated beverage with sugar or a low-calorie sweetener will top off your snack delightfully. Isn't it nice that such delicious foods and beverages are available to satisfy your between-meal hunger and thirst?

Unfortunately, it is not nice for my food-sensitive patients. All the snacks I mentioned are prohibited by our diet because they are high in sugar, MSG, the citric acids, or low-calorie sweeteners.

The reason for the prohibition is not some mean-spirited desire to rob our patients of the satisfaction these snacks provide but to rob these food chemicals of their ability to cause headaches, stuffiness, fuzzy thinking, and all the other ailments that strike our patients. We are trading good taste for good health.

What Can Our Patients Eat for Snacks?

Let's examine some snacks for the food-sensitive person so he or she knows what foods and beverages are acceptable on our diet. As always, if you do not tolerate any individual foods or beverages we recommend, don't eat them.

Beverages

Although there are alternatives for prohibited foods that can satisfy the snack attack, there are few alternatives for the beverages we enjoy and even crave—the highly sweetened or low-calorie carbonated and noncarbonated beverages. Even though my patients enjoy the taste of these beverages, they do not enjoy the distress they cause. Instead, my patients must choose coffee, tea, water, or milk. And they must avoid the excess caffeine of too much coffee and tea.

Sometimes the eating urge is a mistaken interpretation of a thirst signal—the body is really asking for water and not for food. Perhaps this is a common mistake and one of the reasons so many diets specify large amounts of water each day. Therefore, when seized by the desire to snack, first try satisfying it by drinking a glass of water.

Those who must avoid sweetened and fruity beverages will find it handy (and a partial substitute for the sodas we all enjoy) to pour a glass of carbonated mineral water, plain and not flavored. It quiets the desire for a beverage with citrus and sugar, a desire whose fulfillment would later be regretted.

Light Snacks

Often our craving for between-meal foods is more a desire to chew something than a desire to load our stomachs with high-calorie food. If water does not satisfy the snack attack, consider celery and carrots—their crunchy taste may satisfy the desire to chew while at the same time supplying nourishment, vitamins, and minerals without a heavy calorie load.

Apples and pears may also satisfy between meal hunger. Most of our patients can eat these nutritious fruits without provoking allergy symptoms. Another handy way to snack is to keep a container of cantaloupe, honeydew, or watermelon pieces stored in the refrigerator. A dish of these red, yellow, or green fruits is as tasty as it is colorful.

Heavier Snacks

If a light snack will not satisfy the between-meal hunger pangs, here's where all the various breads can come in handy. If they are free of raisins and sugar, they can be eaten freely. If you tolerate peanut butter, spread some on a slice of bread, but first read the label to be sure it is low in sugar and free of other problem ingredients.

Sometimes a slice of acceptable sandwich meat will strike your fancy, perhaps with a glass of milk. Or you might microwave some breakfast sausage you have already precooked and stored in the freezer. A small piece of that chicken you cooked and froze may be just the right thing to appeal to your snack-hungry palate.

As you search for foods to tide you over until the next meal, don't forget the many varieties of crackers. Look for those crackers you bought last week, the ones free of MSG flavorings. Hopefully you purchased a brand low in or free of sugar, such as Nabisco Triscuits (the wheat and bran variety looks good to me) or Kavli Norwegian crispbread, an all-natural cracker made with whole-grain wheat, rye, water, and salt. Don't top them with cheese—eat them plain or with butter, margarine, or peanut butter.

Every time I think of crackers, I think of the number of brands with sugar listed second or third on the label. Crackers are not the only foods with small amounts of sugar; many other foods also contain sugar. This worries me. If my patients eat enough of these foods, they will accumulate significant amounts of dietary refined sugar.

That's why I hesitate to mention the sugared crackers here. An exception may be Sunshine Krispy Original Saltine Crackers, which lists sugar in the sixth position on the list of ingredients (I hope means the quantity is small).

Although the snacks we discussed will satisfy your hunger, sometimes you would rather enjoy a crunchy chip snack. Regretfully, if you are sensitive to the food chemicals we are discussing, potato chips are not for you. But how about a plain corn chip such as Old Dutch Restaurante Style Tortilla Chips or Deli Tostados? Or Frito-Lay Sun Chips, Original Flavor, with corn and other grains (sugar is listed sixth on the label)? Although many of my patients suffer discomfort from corn, they may tolerate the corn in these chips. And for those who need to go easy on fat, why not try the new low-salt pretzels?

One last snack suggestion—pour a small amount of sunflower seeds (free of MSG flavoring) into a bowl and prop your feet up in front of the TV. Enjoy the tube while you savor the sunflower seeds' delicious, crunchy taste.

Dining Out

Every day of our lives we experience annoyance and inconvenience. Maybe an important goal eludes us, a project
fails, or perhaps a silly squabble erupts with a friend or
family member. We don't need problems such as a splitting
headache that threatens to tear apart our head as it ruins
our day. We don't need a churning stomach that forces us
to seek the restroom at a time of great embarrassment. Even
though we do not need—nor do we seek—these aggravating afflictions, we often face them when we go to a nice
restaurant for a fine meal.

This need not be so. People with food allergy can eat at
a restaurant and enjoy the meal, smiling and laughing in
the pleasant companionship of their fellow diners. They
can leave the restaurant with happy memories of sharing a
satisfying meal with good friends and feel as healthy as
those who have no food allergy. To do this, they need only
understand their food allergy and eat and drink foods and
beverages they tolerate.

I remember a patient I treated many years ago whose
story awakened these thoughts in my mind. She had her
share of everyday worries. She did not need the extra trou-

bles brought on by her diet. However, her diet caused great distress, and my attempt to treat this patient was one of the first experiences that turned my attention to food allergy. It made me wish I knew enough about foods to tell her how to dine without regret.

Marlene's Story

It happened years ago but, as with so many other significant events, the memory of my encounter with Marlene remains as clear as if it happened yesterday. I shall never forget it.

When we met, I found Marlene to be a pleasant young woman and mother of three small children. Like so many of my patients, she suffered from many allergic illnesses, and hers included headaches, intermittent hives, and spring and fall hay fever. There was one symptom that was worse then the others, however, and it was enormously embarrassing. As she told me about it, our conversation went something like this.

"Marlene, do you have any trouble with food allergy?" I asked, as I reviewed the various illnesses that brought her to see me.

"Yes, I do have problems with foods, especially when I eat at a restaurant," she answered with a look on her face that convinced me she was reluctant to tell me about it.

"What's the problem, Marlene?"

"It's so embarrassing, Dr. Walsh," she said with a frown. "Having three little children, my husband and I seldom go out to eat, so when we do, it's really a major event, and we look forward to the evening with great anticipation. We usually invite good friends and combine dinner with a show. But we have to go to dinner an hour early because, after I eat, I have to spend an hour in the restroom with terrible diarrhea. I'm embarrassed, my husband is embarrassed, and I'm sure our friends think I'm peculiar."

I understood why Marlene was reluctant to tell me her story—her embarrassment made it difficult for her to discuss what she was going through, even with me. I suspect she worried that I too would think she was peculiar. But I didn't. I saw how this food reaction was putting a strain on her marriage and interfering cruelly with her limited time with friends. For her it was devastating.

At that time, although I sympathized with her, I couldn't help her because my knowledge of food allergy was too limited to know which foods were causing her distress. In retrospect, after treating so many patients with similar diarrheas, I know that the foods causing her diarrhea were those carrying the chemicals that my food-sensitive patients must avoid.

Avoiding the Foods and Beverages That Cause Illness

When my patients or I eat in a restaurant, we must be alert to the foods and beverages that turn the happy enjoyment of an excellent meal into unhappy post-meal pain and discomfort. Some of the foods and beverages that do this are easy to recognize. However, because we like them, we find them hard to avoid. (We need real will power to progress from recognition to avoidance.) Others are hard to avoid because they are hard to recognize—we may not be aware they are in our food.

These hard-to-recognize foods and beverages will be discussed later; for now, let's look those that are easy to recognize.

REFINED SUGAR. If it tastes sweet it is sweet, and probably loaded with refined sugar. Examples such as sweet rolls, sweet sauces, coffee with sugar, syrup, sweet carbonated beverages, pies, cakes, ice cream, cookies, and other treats spring quickly to mind. My food-sensitive patients should not eat or drink these foods and beverages.

LOW-CALORIE SWEETENERS. Our main contact with these chemicals are low-calorie carbonated beverages and those little packets for sweetening coffee or tea. My patients should pass them by.

CITRUS. My patients should recognize foods and beverages containing high levels of citrus as readily as they recognize those loaded with refined sugar—as sugar tastes sweet, citrus and its sister acids taste fruity. Both citrus and sugar are easily identifiable and exceedingly delicious flavors. Why did the angelic imp of allergy load these chemicals with such delightful taste and such atrocious consequences? Neither I nor those affected by these food additives have the answer.

In the restaurant, citrus will be found in the breakfast juice, in the fruit plate that includes oranges or grapefruit, and in foods and beverages flavored with lime or lemon juice. Many sauces and salad dressings contain citrus—ask your waitress or waiter about the ingredients of the sauce or salad dressing before ordering it.

Expect to find citrus in the jelly or jam-like spreads used on bread. Also expect to find it in the many desserts, candies, and carbonated and noncarbonated beverages that have a delectable fruity flavor—here it is usually accompanied by refined sugar. My patients must either refuse these appealing treats or pass them on to a companion who can eat and drink them without pain and discomfort.

Harder to Recognize—Monosodium Glutamate (MSG)

MSG hides under many disguises in a restaurant meal, and aiding its concealment are three factors: (1) It is generally recognized as safe; (2) it can be added by the cook in many forms; (3) it is present in high levels naturally in many foods

IT IS GENERALLY RECOGNIZED AS SAFE. Every cook worth his or her salary wants to prepare an excellent meal for the restaurant's patrons. One method of adding delectable flavor to a meal is to add the delicious flavoring agents and seasonings that contain MSG. (There is no question in my mind that MSG is a superlative flavoring agent; I can usually detect its presence in a meal because of the excellent flavor of the food I am eating.) Expect it in any meat or fish preparation. Expect it in soups where its flavor helps bring a taste of extra robustness. Croutons also contain it for the same reason.

The chef who adds MSG to a meal harbors no malicious desire to harm his patrons. The opposite is true. The chef would never use an additive in the meal if he even suspected that it caused harm. And there is no reason for the chef to suspect MSG; it sits proudly on the FDA's list of the safest food ingredients, the "generally recognized as safe (GRAS)" list.

Therefore, because the chef might not regard MSG as capable of causing distressing symptoms to his patrons, he will probably not take pains to clearly indicate its presence in the food he prepares. His patrons must realize that it is their responsibility to ask about MSG, so they can be sure the food they eat does not contain this flavoring agent.

IT CAN BE ADDED BY THE COOK IN MANY FORMS. Many seasonings and flavorings contain MSG, and unless a chef is especially knowledgeable about the contents of the flavorings and seasonings he uses, he may be using one of these flavorings without knowing it contains MSG. This is not surprising. The MSG content is high in seasonings containing the following ingredients: monosodium glutamate, MSG, hydrolyzed vegetable protein, autolyzed yeast extract, yeast extract, sodium and calcium caseinate, and even cheese and various forms of natural flavorings or natural flavor. With each of these products, the chef can deliver significant quantities of MSG to his patron's meal. I often wonder if the chef who prepares my meal knows how much MSG it contains.

I admit I compound this uncertainty—I am not the brave type who calls for the chef and asks about the MSG content of the food. I ask the waitress or waiter, who then asks the chef, allowing more chance for confusion, especially as the serving person may not know anything about

that strange chemical called MSG and may forget the name
before he or she talks to the chef.

IT IS PRESENT IN HIGH LEVELS NATURALLY IN MANY
FOODS. Avoiding MSG in a restaurant meal is more complicated than just asking the waitress if the chef uses it in meal
preparation. As we discussed before, MSG is found in
many foods naturally. Unless you remember this and avoid
these foods, you may be eating a meal with too much MSG.

Tomatoes not only contain citrus, they also contain
MSG. Corn also contains it, but corn separated from the cob
before boiling should be tolerated. Mushrooms have it, as
do many preparations made with seaweed or kelp (which
are algae). Any fermented or aged food can contain
MSG—well-aged cheese has surprisingly high levels of
MSG, as does soy sauce. My patients must be careful that
their meal does not contain these foods.

Choosing a Meal at a Restaurant

We looked at the restaurant foods and beverages with
problem ingredients. Now let's try to answer the question
my patients ask when they go to a restaurant. What can
they eat?

Imagine yourself in their place. You struggled hard
through the week, whether caring for the children at home,
trying your best at work, or studying diligently at school.
Like a boxer in a prize fight, you fought your best and you
want your reward—a nice meal by yourself, with your family, or with good friends. A post-meal throbbing headache,
aching stomach, or itching skin is not your goal. None of
these qualify as much of a prize.

You do not need to suffer these distressing symptoms.
You can leave the restaurant with your hunger satisfied and
with the knowledge that no pain and discomfort will spoil
your enjoyment. You can feel as healthy as those who do
not share your food sensitivities.

To avoid pain and discomfort, you must select your meal carefully. Don't feel alone in this. I and many other people must also be careful of what we order from the menu because we are also susceptible to the untoward effects of these chemicals. Perhaps some of the things I have learned may help you order wisely and feel good after the meal.

BREAKFAST. For me, breakfast is easy to order. I often order pancakes and an egg, sunny side up. Because of its sugar content, I do not use syrup, but I like to top the pancakes with something, so I place the egg on top of the pancakes and add salt and pepper. This makes a very satisfying combination.

Another breakfast I order is oatmeal or Cream of Wheat, perhaps with a side order of well-cooked bacon and a banana or a slice of melon. No sausage, as it may be flavored with MSG. Some of the dry breakfast cereals, low in refined sugar, would also be acceptable, although I seldom order them.

Sometimes breakfast is served cafeteria-style, where a large selection of breakfast food is available. If there are fish selections, cooked without sauce or breading (which may contain MSG), I load my plate. I enjoy fish. Next I look for the fruit plate and slowly, one by one, load my plate with watermelon and other melon slices while avoiding strawberries and pineapple. I skip the juice and use water or skim milk for my beverage.

For the meat course, I choose bacon or other sliced meats, free of sauce and breading. Sauces and breadings may contain MSG. Someday I hope I will be able to choose foods prepared in sauce or breaded foods. One of my patients is chief of catering at a large and famous hotel in St. Paul—she tells me her catering service does not use MSG for seasoning their meals. Although I believe the public concern about MSG has prompted many food preparers to stop using this additive when they serve breakfast to large groups, I still avoid sauces and breading that may contain it. I don't know which preparers are still using this seasoning, or one that is not pure MSG but contains MSG in large quantities.

The day may come when, as we puzzle over which dishes to choose, we see a little sign telling us which selections contain MSG and which do not. That sign would be most helpful and deeply appreciated.

LUNCH AND DINNER. For me, the problems of food selection in a restaurant tend to be similar at both lunch and dinner, so let's examine the noon and evening meals together.

At both meals, as I peruse the menu, I look for main courses that are simply prepared. I immediately eliminate from consideration all meat, poultry, and fish prepared in sauces and choose a simply processed slice of meat such as a steak, asking the waitress to make sure the chef adds no seasoning. By asking for no seasoning instead of asking for no MSG, I believe I am dodging the need to teach the waitress about MSG and all the seasonings in which it may be found. No seasoning means no MSG, and this simple instruction also means no confused waitress trying to tell the chef not to add that strange seasoning, the name of which she forgot on the way to the kitchen.

Don't assume that because a restaurant is expensive, it does not use MSG to season its steaks. I have made this mistake. I have been in excellent, expensive restaurants where I assumed the steak was so good the chef would not add seasoning. That naive thought turned out to be wrong. MSG was routinely used without any warning on the menu.

On two occasions I discovered this after the steak was served and had to send it back. Because I forgot to ask when I ordered the meal, I felt like a fool, but each time, in spite of this guilty feeling, I sent back the steak. Of course, I was apologetic, but I was also irritated. Why do they add MSG and not tell the patron? (Because the chef does not realize it causes pain and discomfort for people like me.)

If I order fish, I make sure it is prepared without sauces and seasonings. An herb-butter preparation is fine, as are almonds, and both impart a great flavor to the fish.

Salads are a problem. I have learned to eat salad without dressing, and I even find it enjoyable (it took me three years to get used to the taste). Because vinegar is a fermented product, it may contain some quantity of MSG. However, if the food-allergic diner finds a salad without dressing distasteful, vinegar and oil are probably the safest. Be sure the vinegar is white vinegar made from grains and not any of the vinegars made from wine or cider, which contain citric and tartaric acids.

Avoid all salad dressings with tomatoes, cheese, citrus juices, and sugar. Unfortunately, that includes almost all dressings other than oil and vinegar.

At a cafeteria-type lunch or dinner, follow the advice we discussed for a cafeteria-style breakfast. Confine your fruit to apples, pears, bananas, melons, and peaches Lettuce, carrots, celery, onions, ripe olives, beans, sunflower seeds, eggs, and cole slaw are acceptable for a salad. In any pasta dish, examine the dressing for a crumbly appearance—it is probably aged cheese that has been added to enhance the flavor. Aged cheese is naturally high in MSG, because fermentation breaks the milk protein of the cheese into its component amino acids, releasing MSG.

If you must have a dish prepared in a sauce, ask the waiter, waitress, or chef if it contains wine or MSG, or any seasoning with MSG (and hope whoever you ask knows the many different names of the seasonings that contain MSG). To be safe, and if the choice is available, select a meat or fish that is sliced by the chef while you wait

What if you are invited to a restaurant meal where the menu is set and you cannot choose your own food? Do what I do. Eat beforehand. Then, if the food contains the dietary chemicals I must avoid, I eat only part of the meal and tell anyone who notices that I am not hungry. It's the truth. Because of my prior meal, I'm *not* hungry. (Eating beforehand prevents my stomach from overruling my head.)

Reflections

My patients *can* enjoy a meal in a restaurant. Yes, their choices are limited. Yes, they have to abstain from some of the most delicious selections on the menu. But when the meal is finished, they won't suffer food allergy's painful symptoms. They will avoid its headaches and cramping abdominal pains. Their skin will not itch, their noses will not block, they will not see their bathroom scales groan under the bloated water weight, and their thinking will not be slowed by the foods they ate. They won't regret the wonderful feeling that comes from eating properly.

Will my patients follow this advice? Yes, they will. They want to control their health and end the mysterious illnesses that torment their days and nights. They never accepted the idea that their headaches were not treatable, that their abdominal discomfort had no cause, that their tiredness and achiness was all in their heads. They feel better and are determined to do whatever is necessary to continue to feel healthy and free of pain. They will follow this advice.

They can take pride in their determination to eat foods that promote good health. Plus, they gain encouragement because the restaurant owner is noticing this group of patrons that must restrict their choices. Some day I hope they will go the restaurant and see MSG-seasoned meals clearly identified and find far more selections available for those who suffer from foods.

Quick-Service Restaurants

We lead hectic lives, fast-paced and with little time to accomplish all the tasks our multiple roles demand. While we fill the role of employee and breadwinner, we also perform the vitally necessary functions of mother and wife or father and husband. As we fulfill these many responsibilities, it is no wonder that on busy days we find no time to prepare a meal.

For instance, in the short time between work and going to a movie, how do we quiet that persistent inner voice of hunger that demands food? Or, as we plan our child's birthday party, how do we arrange to feed the hungry little gremlins we invite? If we are traveling, where can we grab a quick meal that doesn't slow our headlong race down the road? The answer to each of these questions is found in restaurants we can count on to serve good food quickly.

Because we often need rapidly served meals, a large restaurant industry arose to serve nutritious meals in an efficient and timely manner and in a clean environment. The names of restaurants in this industry—names like McDonald's®, Wendy's Old Fashioned Hamburgers®, and Burger King®—spring readily to mind. They satisfy this need and satisfy it well.

My patients live as hectic a life as any other group of people and often share this need for a rapidly prepared meal. However, for them, satisfying this need raises a troublesome question. When they go to these restaurants, what can they eat?

The Essence of the Problem

Selection of food at any restaurant presents problems for my patients who are sensitive to MSG, low-calorie sweeteners, and excess refined sugar and citrus. To explain how the problem arises, let's pretend we control the destiny of a large chain of quick-service restaurants. Our decisions will make or break the chain, return profits or losses to our investors, and employ thousands of needy workers or force their unemployment. We have a huge responsibility.

This is a competitive industry, and our competitor chains will eagerly pounce on our mistakes. To remain in business, our food must be nutritious, served in a wholesome manner, and taste delicious. This last requirement triggers the problem my patients face.

Each of these restaurant chains, including our hypothetical chain, employs food scientists to prepare menus and advise management. We have our own scientists and we need their advice, especially on the flavorings we use in our food. And for a good reason. If our patrons enjoy the taste of our food, they will return again and again.

Therefore, we listen closely when they discuss the subject of food flavoring. They tell us that the most effective flavoring agent is MSG. Not only is it the most effective flavoring, but it is recognized by the FDA as safe for general use by people of all ages, and this safety is confirmed by many of the scientists who have searched in vain for evidence that MSG causes harm, except in a few, rare cases. They also tell us that we must use it in our food. If we do not, our food will not taste as delicious as that of our competitors who use MSG. Our customers will stay away, our restaurants will fail, and our employees will lose their jobs.

Let's make this even more personal—let's pretend you alone control the restaurants and your decisions mean profits or losses, paychecks or unemployment. Would you use MSG? Yes, you would.

I told you this story for several reasons. One reason is to explain why quick-service restaurants use MSG. Also, to reassure you that using MSG does not mean the restaurant managers unfeelingly disregard your health, they do not. They use MSG only because they think it is safe and wholesome and they do not believe its use will cause you—their customer—any harm. Finally, I told you this story to let you know you will find MSG in quick-service restaurants and you must be constantly vigilant. Order only those foods free of MSG.

Avoiding MSG

Although telling my patients to avoid foods with MSG is easy, avoiding it is hard. The reason is simple. The foods containing MSG must be identified before they can be avoided. The answer to this problem at first seems simple—tell my patients which foods contain this flavoring agent so they can avoid them. Unfortunately, as is so typical in real life, simple answers become complicated when explored.

This became apparent when I discussed MSG in foods with a charming and helpful dietician at McDonald's. At my request, McDonald's sent me the complete list of ingredients of all the foods served at their restaurants. Included in the information was a listing of all their products that contain added MSG and also the products to which McDonald's adds hydrolyzed vegetable protein, which contains MSG. However (isn't life full of *howevers*?), there is still a problem.

The problem arises because McDonald's buys many items of food from different food manufacturers. In the information sent by McDonald's, these foods are included, as are the lists of the ingredients used to prepare them. As I reviewed the information, a troubling ingredient was repeatedly mentioned—natural flavoring.

I explained the FDA's position on the use of MSG in foods in the chapter on MSG. If pure MSG is added, it must be listed. However, if a source of MSG such as hydrolyzed vegetable protein is used, it does not need to be listed on the label and can be identified as natural flavoring. This holds true for autolyzed yeast, yeast extract, and sodium or calcium caseinate, which are all flavoring agents containing MSG. Each of these, if used in high enough quantity, can add enough MSG to my patients' meals to cause distress.

Since McDonald's buys these foods already prepared, and since the composition of the natural flavoring is often a trade secret of the manufacturing company and not known to McDonald's, the dietician did not know if the foods with natural flavoring contain MSG, even though MSG is not acknowledged on the list of ingredients. A concentration of MSG of less then one percent may cause symptoms for my sensitive patients. Since natural flavors may contribute that much MSG to a food selection, my patients may find that eating these foods causes pain and discomfort. When they eat them, they take a great risk.

Which returns us to the question, what foods should my patients avoid at McDonald's and what foods can they order? To try to answer these questions, I spent several hours with the McDonald's brochure, *McDonald's Food: the Facts*, and below I discuss the foods I believe my patients should avoid and also those they can order.

Eating at McDonald's

The following information has been supplied by McDonald's. This same information is available by contacting:

McDonald's Nutrition Information Center
McDonald's Corporation
Oak Brook, Illinois 60521
708/575-FOOD

FOODS AND BEVERAGES MY PATIENTS SHOULD AVOID AT McDONALD'S. Beverages and desserts containing low-calorie sweeteners or large amounts of refined sugar and the citric acids are easy to recognize and therefore easy to avoid (tell that to someone who hungers for a soda and milk shake). We discussed them earlier—the sweet carbonated beverages, juices, syrups, muffins, and various desserts. I will not repeat this information here.

Sauces and dressings taste good because they contain large amounts of refined sugar and/or citrus. My patients have trouble tolerating high levels of sugar and citrus and should avoid both sauces and dressings.

Because MSG is frequently used in food preparation but is also frequently difficult to identify in the foods we eat, we need to look for its presence in all restaurant entrées, including those available at McDonald's. The following foods contain MSG:

FOODS WITH MSG ADDED AS MSG

Breakfast Burrito
Breakfast sausage patty (and sandwiches containing
  sausage):
  Sausage Biscuit
  Sausage Biscuit with Egg
  Sausage McMuffin
  Sausage McMuffin with Egg
  Pizza Sausage
Soups (all of them)

FOODS WITH MSG ADDED AS HYDROLYZED VEGETABLE PROTEIN

Big Mac Sauce

Certain food selections at McDonald's may contain MSG. They are supplied to McDonald's by food manufacturing companies, and these foods contain natural flavors, natural flavoring, or seasoning. Since the composition of the various natural flavorings used in preparing these foods is not specified, they may or may not contain MSG. If they do, the MSG was added in the form of hydrolyzed vegetable protein, autolyzed yeast or yeast extract, sodium or calcium caseinate, or one of the foods with naturally high quantities of MSG. Then, the presence of MSG does not need to be listed in the ingredients.

However, although the content of MSG is not listed, the foods can contain enough of this flavoring agent to cause distress to my patients. To avoid this distress, my patients should avoid these foods.

I suspect that the natural flavorings in salad dressings plus meat, fish, and poultry dishes and their accompanying sauces contain MSG. I listed these selections containing natural flavorings in the following list:

FOODS CONTAINING NATURAL FLAVORINGS THAT MAY CONTAIN MSG

McLean Deluxe
Filet-O-Fish Patty
McChicken Patty
Bacon (not Canadian-style bacon)
Chicken McNuggets
Bacon Bits (for salad)
Chicken (for salad)
Fajita Chicken Strips
Hot Mustard Sauce
Barbecue Sauce
Sweet 'N Sour Sauce
Bleu Cheese Salad Dressing
Ranch Salad Dressing
Red French Reduced-Calorie Salad Dressing

Finally, MSG is released by fermentation from protein in the manufacture of cheese and soy sauce. In most cases, the presence of cheese is obvious—such as in a cheeseburger—and is easy to avoid by ordering a hamburger without cheese. Sometimes the presence of cheese is not so obvious, and these cheese-containing foods, plus food containing soy sauce, make up the following list:

FOODS WITH MSG ADDED AS CHEESE OR SOY SAUCE

Croutons (contain dehydrated Romano cheese)
Chef Salad (contains shredded cheese)
Bleu Cheese Salad Dressing
Barbecue Sauce (contains soy sauce)
Sweet 'N Sour Sauce (contains soy sauce)
Red French Reduced Calorie Salad Dressing
  (contains soy sauce)

FOODS AND BEVERAGES MY PATIENTS CAN ORDER AT McDONALD'S. Now I will change focus and indicate the foods and beverages my patients should be able to tolerate. As always, if a patient has an allergic reaction to a particular food recommended on our diet, this food should be avoided.

To help in food selection, I divided the following selections into those ordered for breakfast and those ordered for both lunch and dinner. Although refined sugar is used in some of the products mentioned below, I believe the quantity of sugar should be tolerated by most food-sensitive patients.

FOODS MY PATIENTS SHOULD TOLERATE FOR BREAKFAST

Egg McMuffin (request it without cheese)
Bacon, Egg, and Cheese Biscuit (request it without
  cheese)
Cheerios
Milk or water

FOODS MY PATIENTS SHOULD TOLERATE FOR LUNCH AND DINNER

Hamburger (with pickles, onion, salt, pepper,
  and mustard)
Quarter Pounder (same as above)
Garden Salad (don't eat the tomato)
Side Salad (don't eat the tomato)
Lite Vinaigrette Salad Dressing (use very little—sugar is
  the third ingredient listed)
Milk or water

Eating at Wendy's

For my food-sensitive patients, the problems surrounding food selection while visiting Wendy's is similar to the those presented by food selection at McDonald's. Avoiding MSG and low-calorie sweeteners plus excess refined sugar and the acids of the citrus group demands careful food selection in each restaurant chain.

To let you know why certain foods on the McDonald's menu are excluded from the list of acceptable foods, we examined the list of ingredients at length. The same ingredients are found in many of the selections at Wendy's. To prevent this chapter from becoming impossibly long, I will not repeat the reasons for excluding foods with these ingredients. Instead, I will concentrate on the foods my patients should tolerate while eating at Wendy's.

I decided to examine Wendy's food because I have received in the mail, on several occasions, detailed information from Wendy's, including the list of ingredients of the foods served at their restaurants. This impressed me. These voluntary mailings indicate that, like McDonald's, Wendy's cares about the health of its patrons.

The following information has been supplied by Wendy's. This same information is available by contacting:

Consumer Relations Department
Wendy's International
P.O. Box 256
Dublin, Ohio 43017
614/764-6800

I used Wendy's classifications in the following list:

FOODS MY PATIENTS SHOULD TOLERATE AT WENDY'S

Meat/Poultry/Fish
Hamburger Patty—Single, Big Classic
Hamburger Patty—Junior, KIDS' MEAL
Breaded Chicken Breast Fillet
Country Fried Steak

Sandwich Toppings
Bacon
Pickles, dill
Tartar sauce

Salad Dressings
Reduced-Calorie Italian (use very little—contains sugar
  and citrus)
Salad oil

Fresh Salads to Go
Side Salad

Potatoes, Chili, and Nuggets
Saltine crackers
Crispy Chicken Nuggets (contains yeast as second-to-
  last ingredient, so quantity should be small)

Beverages
Coffee
Milk
Water

Garden Spot Salad Bar
Bread sticks
Chow mein noodles
Cottage cheese (small amount—fermented product)
Eggs
Garbanzo beans
Green peas
Olives, black
Peaches
Three-bean salad

Reflections on Eating at Quick-Service Restaurants

The selection of foods my patients can tolerate at quick-service restaurants is limited and omits many delicious choices. This I regret. Perhaps it is some small comfort to my patients to know they are not the only ones forced to choose their meal carefully. I too must choose from this limited selection of foods and avoid many I would love to eat.

There are many fine restaurant chains that I did not review because, if I did, this chapter would be impossibly long. Not reviewing them does not mean I consider them inferior in any way.

Many of the foods listed as acceptable to my patients contain refined sugar, and I hope the sugar is present in small quantities. Even though we try to avoid it, our diet still seems to have as much refined sugar as a forest has wood ticks. My sugar-sensitive patient should remember this when hungering for a refined sugar sweet treat after a meal. Because of all the acceptable foods containing small amounts of sugar, my patient has not eaten a sugar-free meal and does not need to add more sugar to the amount already consumed. The dessert or carbonated beverage may be the excess sugar that brings headaches, abdominal cramps, and other pains and discomforts. Best to forget that sweet treat.

I thought that reviewing two restaurants would serve as a model for every other quick-service restaurant my patients may patronize. Unfortunately, I was wrong. Examination of the acceptable choices at both restaurants showed some differences, mostly due to the fact that MSG or natural flavorings is present in a specific food at one restaurant and not in the same food at the other restaurant. This means my patients will not be able to use this information to determine which foods to select at the restaurants of another chain. I wish this were not so.

Those unacquainted with the suffering of the allergic patient will say that no one will follow this advice. They are wrong. They do not understand the discomfort my patients suffer from food, nor do they understand their determination of to take control of their health and end the symptoms that are such a scourge.

They do not know my patients with daily migraine headaches, whose doctors were unable to stop this terrible pain. Nor do they know my patients with untreatable hives, cramps and diarrhea, and tiredness. They do not realize that my patients did not give up searching for answers and relief.

Now that my patients know these answers, they will not allow foods to harm them. They are brave and determined people; they will follow this advice.

Do I recommend that my patients eat at Wendy's or McDonald's? You bet I do (I have no connection to either chain, nor am I paid by them).

Please believe that those who operate McDonald's, Wendy's, and other quick-service restaurants are just like you and me. They have no desire to serve food that may make my patients sick. If the managers and employees of these restaurants become convinced that MSG, low-calorie sweeteners, and excess sugar and citrus cause trouble for their patrons, they will provide more food selections free of these chemicals.

How will they know? They will know if their patrons carefully select certain foods and avoid others. The power of the consumer is awesome.

Recipes

An Introduction to Felicia Busch

As a diplomate of the American Board of Allergy and Immunology, I am trained in the treatment of patients with food allergy. But being a specialist in treating food-sensitive patients does not mean I am a specialist in the food sciences.

I can diagnose food allergy and instruct my patients to avoid offending foods. However, my specialty training has not prepared me to prescribe a diet with the knowledge and authority possessed by a registered dietician. Only they have the qualifications necessary to ensure meeting nutritional needs while formulating meal plans and menus for people whose health requires a special diet.

Recognizing this limitation, I was delighted when Felicia Busch agreed to put her specialty to work helping my patients. Felicia brings many unique qualifications to this task, not the least of which is that she is an experienced and competent registered dietician.

Felicia's academic credentials are impressive. She obtained a master's degree in public health from the University of Minnesota and a bachelor's degree in dietetics and nutrition from Florida International University. She is a registered member of the American Dietetic Association.

In her professional career, Felicia was employed by the Ramsey County Health Department as Health Promotion Coordinator. She has also held a variety of positions in public health and corporate wellness programs.

Felicia currently serves as a national media spokesperson for the American Dietetic Association, is a past president of the Minnesota Nutritional Council, and is president-elect of the Twin Cities District Dietetic Association.

In 1986 Felicia started her own consulting company, Felicia Busch and Associates, which provides consultation on nutrition and health communications to over 150 corporate and education clients. She appears on numerous radio and television news programs as a nutrition expert and has her own regionally syndicated radio program, "Food for Thought."

As impressive as these credentials are, the most important one for us is that Felicia is an author, and a good one. She has written several chapters for *Personal Nutrition*, a college textbook on nutrition. Many national magazines feature her articles on health and nutrition. All of this experience makes her uniquely qualified to understand the plight of food-sensitive people and to use her skills and knowledge to help guide them on the path to health.

As I mentioned, I was delighted to have someone of her background and ability agree to help guide those patients of mine who must restrict sugar, MSG, citrus, and low-calorie sweeteners. I am sure you will share my sentiment as you learn her approach to a diet that is designed to help my patients feel well.

On the following pages, Felicia provides information on nutrition, shopping tips, menu plans, and recipes to increase our patients' success with using the diet.

What's Left To Eat

By Felicia Busch, M.P.H., R.D.

What's left to eat? I have been asked that question at least a thousand times by patients who have had to make changes in their diets for a variety of reasons. Whether it's food allergy restrictions, a low-cholesterol diet, or a low-sodium diet, the first reaction is to think that there is nothing worth eating left on your list. Try, instead, to focus on all the wonderful foods you have to choose from.

Right now, it's most important to concentrate on the changes in your diet needed to make you feel better. The following dietary guidelines for Americans are the basis of sound eating for healthy adults. Use these guidelines as a model for planning your food choices, but keep in mind that eliminating foods that cause you harm is your main priority now. A balanced diet is something to achieve over time, not overnight.

The Dietary Guidelines for Americans

Eat a variety of foods to get the energy, protein, vitamins, minerals and fiber you need for good health.

Maintain a healthy weight to reduce your chances of having high blood pressure, heart disease, certain cancers, and diabetes.

Choose a diet low in fat, saturated fat, and cholesterol to reduce your risk of heart disease and certain types of cancer. Because fat contains more than twice the calories of other foods, a diet low in fat can help you maintain a healthy weight.

Choose a diet with plenty of vegetables, fruits, and grain products, which provide needed vitamins, minerals, fiber, and complex carbohydrates.

Use sugars only in moderation. A diet with lots of sugars has too many calories and too few nutrients for most people and can help cause tooth decay.

Use salt and sodium only in moderation to help reduce your risk of high blood pressure.

If you drink alcoholic beverages, do so in moderation. Alcoholic beverages supply calories but little or no nutritional value.

Following Through

It has been my experience in over fifteen years as a registered dietician that people with food allergies are more likely to be faithful to their special diets. You will actually feel much better when you eliminate problem foods. And there is nothing like feeling great to help reinforce the benefits of a new way of eating. After the initial anxiety of eliminating or reducing many of your favorite foods, you'll find there are lots of delicious and nutritious foods you can eat that will make you feel good.

It does take extra time and planning to follow any special diet. Budget more time at the grocery store to read food labels. You'll need extra minutes in the kitchen to make some recipes from scratch. Try to keep your kitchen stocked with staples. That way, at the end of a busy day you won't have to worry about what to fix for dinner—you'll have all the basic ingredients on hand.

I find it helpful to sketch out menus a week in advance. You don't have to plan down to the last detail, but a rough idea will help you stay on track. To help you get started I have put together a week's worth of sample menus and recipes that fit the specific requirements of Dr. Walsh's dietary recommendations. Remember that one diet will not work for everyone; each individual has his or her own specific nutrient needs and reactions to foods. Adapt these suggestions to meet your particular needs, adding or subtracting foods as necessary. Bon appétit!

Tips for High-Nutrition Shopping

Any type of dietary limitation requires careful attention to be sure that a wide enough variety of foods is included to guarantee a balanced diet. To choose foods rich in vitamins and minerals consider, the following recommendations:

WHEN BUYING BREADS, GRAINS, RICE, AND PASTA: Choose whole-grain varieties whenever possible; they contain more B Vitamins and fiber than refined products. Read the label of breads to see if whole-grain flour is listed first.

Choose cooked and ready-to-eat cereals with no more than two grams of fat and at least two grams of fiber per serving. Avoid cereals with added sugar.

WHEN BUYING FRUITS AND VEGETABLES: Choose loose leaf lettuce like romaine and endive that contain many nutrients instead of iceberg lettuce with few nutrients.

Choose dark green broccoli and deep orange carrots instead of poorly colored ones. Darkly colored green and yellow vegetables have more vitamins and minerals that lightly colored ones.

Choose fresh fruits and vegetables in season to provide maximum nutrition. When foods are not in season or look inferior in quality, choose plain frozen varieties.

Purchase canned fruits packed in water or juice and drain before using. Eat at least five servings of fruits and vegetables a day for good health.

WHEN BUYING DAIRY PRODUCTS: Choose low-fat and skim milk foods instead of whole milk varieties. Limit your intake of cheese, and choose only plain yogurt. The fermentation process used to manufacture such products releases MSG. Some individuals may not tolerate any cheese or yogurt; others can eat limited amounts.

WHEN BUYING MEAT, POULTRY, AND SEAFOOD: Choose lean, well-trimmed fresh cuts of meat whenever possible. Remove all skin and fat from poultry before cooking. Choose lean ground beef and drain all excess fat while cooking.

Choose fresh or frozen fish and seafood without bread-ing, tuna packed in water. Check canned tuna for added MSG.

Always read the label of processed meats to see if MSG or MSG-containing flavorings are added. Product formula-tions change frequently, so read and check labels each time you buy.

Foods To Keep on Hand

BREADS, GRAIN, RICE, AND CEREALS
(six to eleven servings recommended per day)

Plain white, whole-wheat, and other whole-grain breads
Bagels and English muffins
White and whole-wheat flour
White and whole-wheat flour tortillas
White, brown, and wild rice
Pasta and noodles, assorted shapes and sizes
Oatmeal
Cold cereals (without added sugar)
Hot cereals

VEGETABLES
(three to five servings recommended per day)

Artichokes
Asparagus
Beets
Broccoli, boiled only
Cabbage, boiled only
Carrots
Celery
Corn, cut off the cob and boiled only
Cucumbers
Green beans
Lettuce
Okra
Olives, without pimento
Onion

Parsnips
Radishes
Rutabagas
Squash
Yams, sweet potatoes

FRUITS
(two to four servings recommended per day)

Apples
Bananas
Cantaloupe
Honeydew melon
Peaches
Pears
Nectarines
Watermelon

DAIRY PRODUCTS
(two to three servings recommended per day)

Milk—skim, low-fat or whole

MEATS AND MEAT ALTERNATIVES
(two servings recommended per day)

Beef
Chicken
Fresh pork
Tuna (avoid canned varieties with added MSG)
Turkey

SEASONINGS

Basil
Cinnamon
Garlic powder or salt
Nutmeg
Onion powder or salt
Oregano
Pepper
Salt
Vanilla
White vinegar (do not substitute flavored vinegars)

Suggested Menus

Day 1

BREAKFAST

Scrambled egg
Lean Canadian bacon
Toast with margarine
Cantaloupe slice
Coffee, tea, or milk

LUNCH

Grilled or baked chicken sandwich with lettuce
Carrot and celery sticks
Fresh apple
Milk

DINNER

Meatloaf
Green beans, boiled
Herbed white rice*
Dinner roll with margarine
Milk

Day 2

BREAKFAST

Oatmeal
Bagel with margarine or butter
Coffee, tea, or milk

LUNCH

Spinach salad with oil and white vinegar dressing*
Bacon bits and chopped egg, if desired
Whole-grain bread with margarine
Canned peaches and pear slices, packed in juice and
   drained before eating
Milk

*Recipes included.

DINNER

Pork chop
Cabbage, boiled well
Sweet potato
Rye bread with margarine
Milk

Day 3

BREAKFAST

Puffed cereal
Banana
Toast with margarine
Coffee, tea, or milk

LUNCH

Plain hamburger with lettuce, onion, pickles, and
    mustard (check mustard for MSG)
Side salad, oil and white vinegar dressing*
Apple
Milk

DINNER

Broiled fish
Cooked carrots
Marinated cucumbers*
Dinner roll with margarine
Milk

Day 4

BREAKFAST

French toast
Mashed fruit for topping, made from allowed fruits
Coffee, tea, or milk

*Recipes included.

LUNCH

Burrito made with tortilla filled with ground beef,
    chopped lettuce, and onion
Watermelon chunks or allowable fruit in season
Milk

DINNER

Homemade chicken and noodles*
Beets
Tossed salad with oil and white vinegar dressing*
Milk

Day 5

BREAKFAST

Shredded wheat
Milk
Honeydew melon

LUNCH

Salad Nicoise*
Fruit cup, peaches, pears, apple chunks (rinse if canned)
Milk

DINNER

Steak
Mashed rutabaga with margarine
Broccoli, boiled
Tossed salad with oil and white vinegar dressing*
Milk

Day 6

BREAKFAST

Buttermilk pancakes*
Mashed fruit for topping (from allowed fruits)
Coffee, tea, or milk

*Recipes included.

LUNCH

Pasta Primavera*
Whole-grain bread with margarine
Milk

DINNER

Roast turkey with homemade gravy
Yams or squash
Green beans, boiled
Bread stuffing*
Baking powder biscuits with margarine
Milk

Day 7

BREAKFAST

Banana muffins*
Stewed apples
Coffee, tea, or milk

LUNCH

Roast beef sandwich with lettuce and sprouts
Fresh pear
Pretzels
Milk

DINNER

Oven-baked chicken
Seasoned wild rice*
Corn, cut off the cob and boiled
Dinner roll with margarine
Milk

*Recipes included.

Recipes

Main Dishes

HOMEMADE CHICKEN AND NOODLES

3- to 4-pound chicken
1 pound egg noodles
1 medium onion
1 cup celery, diced
2 tablespoons margarine or butter
1 teaspoon salt
⅛ teaspoon pepper
¼ cup flour
Paprika

Boil chicken in 6 cups water until tender, about 2½ hours. Reserve 4 cups chicken broth. Remove chicken from bones in large pieces. Prepare noodles according to package directions and drain. Sauté onion and celery in margarine until tender; stir in flour and mix well. Combine chicken, noodles, reserved broth, onion, celery, salt, and pepper. Pour into two 2-quart or one very large casserole. Bake uncovered at 350° for 30 minutes. Sprinkle top with paprika. Freeze one casserole for later use, if desired.

MEAT LOAF

1 pound ground beef
¼ cup bread crumbs
½ cup milk
1 egg, beaten
Salt and pepper to taste

Mix all ingredients thoroughly. Shape into loaf and bake at 350° for 1 hour.

PASTA PRIMAVERA

½ pound spaghetti, regular to thin style
2 cups broccoli, boiled
3 large carrots, sliced and cooked
1 cup corn, cut from cob and boiled
⅔ cup olive oil
¼ cup white vinegar (do not substitute flavored vinegars)

$\frac{1}{4}$ cup parsley, chopped
2 tablespoon dried basil (use $\frac{1}{4}$ cup if fresh)
1 clove garlic
$\frac{1}{2}$ teaspoon salt
$\frac{1}{4}$ teaspoon pepper

Cook pasta according to package directions. Rinse in cold water and drain well. In large bowl, combine broccoli, carrots, and corn. Add pasta and toss gently. In blender or food processor, blend oil, vinegar, parsley, basil, garlic, salt, and pepper until smooth. Pour over pasta and toss.

SALAD NICOISE

$\frac{3}{4}$ cup olive oil
$\frac{1}{4}$ cup white vinegar (do not substitute flavored vinegars)
2 tablespoons chopped parsley
Salt and pepper to taste
4 cups mixed salad greens
$\frac{1}{4}$ pound whole green beans, cooked
3 hard-cooked eggs, cut into wedges
$6\frac{3}{4}$-ounce can tuna, drained (check label to be sure MSG is not added)
1 small onion, cut into rings

Combine oil, vinegar, parsley, salt, and pepper. Toss 2 tablespoons dressing over the green beans and marinate 30 minutes. Arrange salad greens on plate. Arrange green beans, eggs, tuna, and onion over greens. Top with dressing or serve on the side.

Side Dishes

BREAD STUFFING

$4\frac{1}{2}$ cups soft bread cubes, not store bought
$\frac{1}{2}$ cup butter or margarine
$\frac{1}{4}$ cup minced onion
2 stalks celery with leaves, chopped
1 teaspoon salt
1 teaspoon sage
$\frac{1}{2}$ teaspoon thyme
$\frac{1}{2}$ teaspoon black pepper

In large skillet, cook and stir onion in butter or margarine until tender. Stir in about one-third of the bread cubes.

Pour bread and onion mixture into bowl and add remaining bread and spices. Mix well. Press into baking dish and bake at 350° for 45 minutes.

SAUSAGE* STUFFING VARIATION: Decrease bread cubes to 4 cups and omit salt. Add ½ pound crumbled cooked sausage.

*Be sure to read entire ingredient list to ensure no MSG has been added to the sausage.

MARINATED CUCUMBERS

2–3 medium cucumbers
1 tablespoon salt
¾ cup white vinegar (do not substitute flavored vinegars)
1 tablespoon sugar*
¼ teaspoon pepper

Wash cucumbers and pat dry. Cut into paper-thin slices. Place slices in a deep bowl and sprinkle every few layers with the 1 tablespoon of salt. Let stand at room temperature for 2 hours. Drain thoroughly. Stir together remaining ingredients and pour over slices. Cover and refrigerate at least 4 hours. Drain cucumbers before serving.

OIL AND VINEGAR DRESSING

⅔ cup salad oil
½ cup white vinegar (do not substitute flavored vinegars)
2 teaspoons dried mustard
1 teaspoon dried basil, crushed
1 teaspoon dried oregano, crushed
½ teaspoon dried dillweed

In screw-top jar, combine all ingredients and shake well to mix. Keep chilled in refrigerator and shake again before serving. Dressing tastes best if allowed to sit at least 24 hours before first use.

SEASONED WILD RICE

1 cup uncooked wild rice
½ cup margarine or butter

4 tablespoons chopped onion
2 stalks celery, chopped
½ teaspoon garlic salt

Wash and rinse dry rice. Place rice in heavy saucepan with 4 cups lightly salted water. Bring to a boil, then cover and simmer for 45 minutes. Uncover and fluff with a fork. Let stand an additional 5 to 10 minutes. Melt margarine in saucepan and sauté onion and celery. Toss garlic, salt, rice, and sautéed vegetables together to mix well.

Breakfast

BASIC MUFFIN BATTER

1 egg
1 cup milk
¼ cup salad oil
2 cups flour
¼ cup sugar*
3 teaspoons baking powder
1 teaspoon salt

Heat oven to 400°. Grease the bottoms of 12 muffin cups or spray with cooking oil. Beat egg, and stir in milk and oil. Mix in remaining ingredients just until flour is moistened. Batter should be lumpy. Fill muffin cup two-thirds full. Bake for 20 to 25 minutes or until golden brown. Immediately remove from pan. Makes 12 muffins.

*The amount of sugar per muffin is just 1 teaspoon. You may choose to decrease the amount even further, but the muffins will lose some of their moistness and texture. Whenever you use sugar in a recipe, be sure to carefully limit additional sugar consumed per day.

VARIETY MUFFINS

APPLE: Stir in 1 cup grated apple and add ½ teaspoon cinnamon. Bake for 25 to 30 minutes.

BANANA: Stir in one large or two small, very ripe, mashed bananas. Add 1 teaspoon of vanilla. Bake for 25 to 30 minutes.

OATMEAL: Decrease white flour to one cup and add one cup oats.

WHOLE WHEAT: Decrease white flour to one cup and add one cup whole-wheat flour. Decrease baking powder to 2 teaspoons.

BUTTERMILK PANCAKES

2 cups sifted flour
1 teaspoon baking soda
1 teaspoon salt
1 tablespoon sugar*
2 eggs
2 cups buttermilk
2 tablespoons margarine, melted

Heat an oiled griddle until hot. Sift together flour, soda, salt, and sugar. In a separate bowl, mix eggs, buttermilk, and margarine. Mix wet and dry ingredients together with spoon until just mixed. Batter will be lumpy. Spoon batter onto griddle and turn when top surface is full of bubbles. Turn only once.

*The amount of sugar per serving of pancakes is less than one teaspoon. You may choose to eliminate the sugar altogether. Whenever you use sugar in a recipe, be sure to carefully limit the total amount of additional sugar consumed per day.

CANTALOUPE COOLER

1 cup cantaloupe, cut into large chunks
½ cup milk, very cold
1 teaspoon vanilla

Whirl all ingredients in blender. Makes a refreshing 12-ounce drink.

Bibliography

Abelson, P. H., Butz, E., and Snyder, S. H. *Neuroscience.* Washington, D.C.: American Association for the Advancement of Science, 1985.

Allen, D. H., Delohery, J., and Baker, G. "Monosodium L-Glutamate Induced Asthma," *Journal of Allergy and Clinical Immunology,* Vol. 80, 1987: pp. 530–7.

Allstetter, B., "Cheating Brain Death," *Discover,* Vol. 12, No. 8, August 1991: p. 24.

Baringa, M., "Amino Acids: How Much Is Too Much?" *Science,* Vol. 247, January 5, 1990: pp. 20–22.

Bigelow, W. D., and Dunbar, P. B. "The Acid Content of Fruits," *Journal of Industrial and Engineering Chemistry,* Vol. 9, No. 8, August 1917: pp. 762–767.

Choi, D. W., "Amyotrophic Lateral Sclerosis and Glutamate—Too Much of a Good Thing?" *The New England Journal of Medicine,* Vol. 326, No. 22, May 28, 1992: pp. 1493–1495.

Costa, E., and Greengard, P. *Advances in Biochemical Psychopharmacology, Volume 27, Glutamate as a Neurotransmitter.* New York: Raven Press, 1981.

Ebert, A. G. Letters to the Editor, *Journal of Asthma*, Vol. 20, No. 2, 1983: pp. 161–3.

Ensminger, A. H., Ensminger, M. E., Konland, E. K., and Robson, J. R. K. *Foods and Nutrition Encyclopedia*. Clovis, California: Pegus Press, 1983.

Fernandez-Flores, E., Kline, D. A., Johnson, A. R., and Leber, B. L. "Quantitative and Qualitative TLC Analysis of Free Amino Acids in Fruits and Fruit Juices," *Journal of the Association of Official Analytical Chemists*, Vol. 53, No. 6, 1970: pp. 1203–8.

Filer, L. J., Garattini, S., Kare, M. R., Reynolds, W. A., and Wurtman, R. J. (eds.) *Glutamic Acid: Advances in Biochemistry and Physiology*. New York: Raven Press, 1979.

Guidotti, A. *Fidia Research Foundation Symposium Series, Volume 4, Neurotoxicity of Excitatory Amino Acids*. New York: Raven Press, 1990.

Hac, L. R., Long, M. L., and Blish, M. J. "The Occurrence of Free L-Glutamic Acid in Various Foods," *Food Technology*, October 1949: pp. 351–4.

Kliewer, W. M. "Free Amino Acids and Other Nitrogenous Substances of Table Grape Varieties," *Journal of Food Science*, Vol. 34, 1969: pp. 274–8.

Leon, A. S., Hunninghake, D. B., Bell, C., Rassin, D. K., and Tephly, T. R. "Safety of Long-Term Large Doses of Aspartame," *Archives of Internal Medicine*, Vol. 149, October 1989: pp. 2318–24.

Maeda, S., Egushi, S., and Sasaki, H. "The Free L-Glutamic Acid Content of Foods (Report No. 2)," *Journal of Home Economics*, Vol. 12, No. 2, 1969: pp. 105–6.

Olney, J. W. "Brain Lesions, Obesity, and Other Disturbances in Mice Treated with Monosodium Glutamate," *Science*, Vol. 164, May 9, 1969: pp. 119–21.

Olney, J. W. "Brain Damage in Infant Mice Following Oral Intake of Glutamate, Aspartate, or Cysteine," *Nature*, Vol. 227, August 8, 1970: pp. 609–11.

Potenza, D. P., and El-Mallakh, R. S. "Aspartame: Clinical Update," *Connecticut Medicine*, Vol. 53, No. 7, July 1989: pp. 395–400.

Reinhardt, D., and Schmidt, E. *Nestle Nutrition Workshop Series, Volume 17, Food Allergy*. New York: Raven Press, 1988.

Robinson, A. L., "Neurotransmitters Regulate Growth Cones," *Science*, Vol. 234, December 12, 1986: pp. 1325–6.

Rothstein, J. D., Martin, L. J., and Kuncl, R. W., "Decreased Glutamate Transport by the Brain and Spinal Cord in Amyotrophic Lateral Sclerosis," *The New England Journal of Medicine*, Vol. 325, No. 22, May 28, 1992: pp. 1464–1468.

Saravis, S., Schachar, R., Zlotkin, S., Leiter, L. A., and Anderson, G. H. "Aspartame: Effects on Learning, Behavior, and Mood," *Pediatrics*, Vol. 86, No. 1, July 1990: pp. 75–83.

Scopp, A. L. "MSG and Hydrolyzed Vegetable Protein Induced Headache: Review and Case Studies," *Headache*, Vol. 31, No. 2, February 1991: pp. 107–10.

Souci, S. W., Fachmann, W., and Kraut, H. *Food Composition and Nutrition Tables 1986/87*. Stuttgart, Germany: Wissenschaftliche Verlagsgesellshaft GmbH, 1986.

SteginK, L. D., Filer, L. J. *Aspartame: Physiology and Biochemistry*. New Yor, and Basel: Marcel Dekker, Inc., 1984.

Swan, G. F. Letters to the Editor, *Journal of Asthma*, Vol. 20, No. 2, 1983: pp. 159–61.

U.S. Department of Agriculture, Food and Drug Administration, "Monosodium Glutamate (MSG)," *FDA Backgrounder*, October 1991.

Wilkin, J. K., "Does Monosodium Glutamate Cause Flushing (Or Merely 'Glutamania')?" *Journal of the American Academy of Dermatology*, Vol. 15, 1986: pp. 225–30.

Wurtman, R. J., and Wurtman, J. J. *Nutrition and the Brain, Volume 6, Physiological and Behavioral Effects of Food Constituents*. New York: Raven Press, 1983.

Yost, D. A. "Clinical Safety of Aspartame," *American Family Physician*, Vol. 39, No. 2, February 1989: pp. 201–6.

Zautcke, J. L., Schwartz, J. A., and Mueller, E. J. "Chinese Restaurant Syndrome: A Review," *Annals of Emergency Medicine*, Vol. 15, No. 10, October 1986: pp. 1210–13.

Index